PHARMACY TECHNICIAN LABORATORY MANUAL

Sandeep Bansal, PT, MPA
Pharmacy Technician Instructor

JONES AND BARTLETT PUBLISHERS

Sudbury, Massachusetts

BOSTON   TORONTO   LONDON   SINGAPORE

World Headquarters

Jones and Bartlett Publishers
40 Tall Pine Drive
Sudbury, MA 01776
978-443-5000
info@jbpub.com
www.jbpub.com

Jones and Bartlett Publishers
Canada
6339 Ormindale Way
Mississauga, Ontario L5V 1J2
Canada

Jones and Bartlett Publishers
International
Barb House, Barb Mews
London W6 7PA
United Kingdom

Jones and Bartlett's books and products are available through most bookstores and online booksellers. To contact Jones and Bartlett Publishers directly, call 800-832-0034, fax 978-443-8000, or visit our website, www.jbpub.com.

Substantial discounts on bulk quantities of Jones and Bartlett's publications are available to corporations, professional associations, and other qualified organizations. For details and specific discount information, contact the special sales department at Jones and Bartlett via the above contact information or send an email to specialsales@jbpub.com.

The authors, editor, and publisher have made every effort to provide accurate information. However, they are not responsible for errors, omissions, or for any outcomes related to the use of the contents of this book and take no responsibility for the use of the products and procedures described. Treatments and side effects described in this book may not be applicable to all people; likewise, some people may require a dose or experience a side effect that is not described herein. Drugs and medical devices are discussed that may have limited availability controlled by the Food and Drug Administration (FDA) for use only in a research study or clinical trial. Research, clinical practice, and government regulations often change the accepted standard in this field. When consideration is being given to use of any drug in the clinical setting, the health care provider or reader is responsible for determining FDA status of the drug, reading the package insert, and reviewing prescribing information for the most up-to-date recommendations on dose, precautions, and contraindications, and determining the appropriate usage for the product. This is especially important in the case of drugs that are new or seldom used.

Production Credits
Publisher: David Cella
Production Director: Amy Rose
Associate Editor: Maro Gartside
Senior Production Editor: Renée Sekerak
Senior Production Editor: Tracey Chapman
Associate Production Editor: Kate Stein
Senior Marketing Manager: Barb Bartoszek
Associate Marketing Manager: Lisa Gordon
Manufacturing and Inventory Control Supervisor: Amy Bacus
Composition: Publishers' Design & Production Services, Inc.
Art: Publishers' Design & Production Services, Inc.
Assistant Photo Researcher: Bridget Kane
Cover Design: Anne Spencer
Cover Image: © Jones and Bartlett Publishers. Courtesy of Maryland Institute for Emergency Medical Services Systems.
Printing and Binding: Courier Stoughton
Cover Printing: Courier Stoughton

ISBN 978-0-7637-5660-4

6048

Printed in the United States of America
13 12 11 10 09   10 9 8 7 6 5 4 3 2 1

Contents

Acknowledgments

To my parents for their genes, my husband Charanjeet for his love, and Hummi, Kim, Raji, and Nadia
for their friendship and support.

Thank you to Christine, Belal, and Don for their time and effort.

Last but not least, to my grandparents.

And I thank Him.

Words of wisdom:

"Life is not a journey to the grave with intentions of arriving safely in a pretty well-preserved body, but rather
to skid in broadside, thoroughly used up, totally worn out and loudly proclaiming . . . WOW! What a ride!"

~Unknown~

"When it comes to the future, there are three kinds of people: those who let it happen, those who make it
happen, and those who wonder what happened."

~John M. Richardson~

Contributors

Donald Willis is currently the pharmacy manager of four hospitals at California Pacific Medical Center in San Francisco, California. Mr. Willis has been a pharmacy technician for 34 years. He received his BA and pharmacy technician training at Duke University. He resides in Oakland, California.

Belal A. Kaifi is finishing his doctoral degree at the University of San Francisco, where he is studying Organizational Leadership. His undergraduate- and graduate-level degrees are in Human Resource Management and Strategic Management. Mr. Kaifi currently teaches at Franklin University and Western Career College and is affiliated with the Phi Delta Kappa Society at the University of San Francisco, the National Honor Society for Public Administration, and the Pi Alpha Alpha Honor Society at California State University. He is grateful to Dr. Herda, Dr. Younos, Dr. Mitchell, and Dr. Gerrard for their ongoing support.

Christine Perez is a licensed Pharmacy Technician with 10 years of experience.

Preface

Welcome to the pharmacy technician profession. There are many areas in the healthcare field where opportunities for pharmacy technicians are growing. These include the biotech industry, hospital pharmacy, community pharmacy, and pharmacy chain stores, to mention a few. Duties traditionally performed by the pharmacist are now being performed by the technician, expanding the role and education of technicians.

As a former student, I have designed this lab manual with the student in mind. The exercises and activities reflect the didactic education learned in the classroom. As an instructor, I have designed this lab manual to complement classroom instruction and help the students implement their teachings.

Self-Evaluation

One crucial part of being a pharmacy technician is to realize your capabilities. As a pharmacy technician it is vital to be empathetic to the patients and to have excellent communication skills. This exercise is probably the easiest lab in this book, and the one filled with the most self-awareness.

You must answer these questions with thought, and please, take your time.

1. Why do I, _____ want to be in the health field?

_____

_____

_____

_____

_____

_____

2. Why do I want to be a pharmacy technician?

_____

_____

_____

_____

_____

_____

_____

3. Why would I make an excellent pharmacy technician?

_____

_____

_____

_____

_____

_____

4. What would make me a bad pharmacy technician? (What are your weaknesses that need to be worked on? Lateness, attitude, etc.)

_____

_____

_____

_____

_____

_____

_____

These questions are those that ALL individuals who enter the health field must ask themselves regardless of what field they are entering. If you know your weaknesses and strengths, your instructor can help you to further build on your strengths as well as work on your weaknesses.

Lab 1: Terminology

OBJECTIVE

After completion of this exercise, the student will understand the terminology used to define basic pharmacology.

INSTRUCTIONS

Using your textbook or other reference materials available in the classroom, define each of the following terms.

Plants: _____

_____

_____

Animals: _____

_____

_____

Chemical synthesis: _____

_____

_____

Drug: _____

_____

_____

Therapeutic effect: _____

_____

_____

Drug indication: _____

_____

_____

Contraindications: _____

_____

_____

Side effects: _____

_____

_____

Adverse effects: _____

_____

_____

Toxic effects: _____

_____

_____

Site of action: _____

_____

_____

Mechanism of action: _____

_____

_____

Receptor site: _____

_____

_____

Agonist: _____

_____

_____

Antagonist: _____

_____

_____

Dose-response curve:_____

_____

_____

Time-response curve: _____

_____

_____

ED50: _____

_____

_____

LD50: _____

_____

_____

Therapeutic index: _____

_____

_____

Chemical name: _____

_____

_____

Generic name: _____

_____

_____

Trade name: _____

_____

_____

Drug forms: _____

_____

_____

Routes of administration: _____

_____

_____

Drug absorption: _____

_____

_____

Drug distribution: _____

_____

_____

Drug metabolism:_____

_____

_____

Drug elimination:_____

_____

_____

Pediatric drug considerations:_____

_____

_____

Factors of individual variation: _____

_____

_____

Drug interactions: _____

_____

_____

Drug Abuse Terminology

Dependence: _____

_____

_____

Addiction: _____

_____

_____

Tolerance: _____

_____

_____

Lab 2: Pharmacy Technician Job Description

OBJECTIVE

After completion of this exercise, the student will understand the position of a pharmacy technician through research of job descriptions.

INSTRUCTIONS

You have just become a pharmacist, but you have a dilemma. You need help. You have a brilliant idea and create a pharmacy technician position. As a pharmacist you are responsible for creating chemicals to make people feel better and have no time for "other business." Working individually or as a group, create a job description of a pharmacy technician. As a hiring manager you need to include the characteristics a person needs to work in a pharmacy. Visit pharmacies, speak with pharmacists, or simply observe pharmacies in action to complete this lab excercise. Your job description will be presented orally at the end of class.

_____

_____

_____

_____

_____

_____

_____

_____

_____

_____

_____

_____

_____

Lab 3: History of Pharmacy

OBJECTIVE

By completing this exercise, the student will learn about the different people who have contributed to the pharmacy profession.

INSTRUCTIONS

The pharmacy profession began thousands of years ago by what some civilizations called medicine men and shamans. In this lab exercise you will complete research on some of the famous—and not so famous—people who contributed to the creation of illegal and legal drugs, as well as the founder of pharmacology. After conducting your research, write a 1–2 page paper answering the following topic:

Choose 3 of the following people or groups and explain how they contributed to the pharmacy/drug profession. Also consider Roman and Arabian influences on the profession.

1. German chemist Friedrich Gaedcke
2. Saint healers
3. Bayer Pharmaceutical
4. Hippocrates
5. Galen
6. Dioscorides
7. Pythagoras
8. Artemidorus
9. Asclepius
10. Chiron and Achilles
11. Apollo

12. Ebers Papyrus
13. Paracelsus
14. Claude Bernard
15. Sir Frederick Banting & Charles Best
16. Gerhardt Domagk
17. Sir Alexander Fleming
18. Oswald Schmiedeberg
19. Dr. Albert Hoffmann
20. Chief Justice William H. Rehnquist
21. Justice Sandra Day O'Connor

Lab 4: Creating DEA Numbers

OBJECTIVE

By completing this exercise, the student will learn how to calculate DEA numbers in order to verify them on prescriptions.

EXERCISE 1

For the following physicians, create DEA numbers. Write the appropriate DEA number for each physician in the prescriptions throughout the manual.

Dr. Bansal, Sandeep _____

Dr. Phull, Hardeep _____

Dr. Mundian, Kim _____

Dr. Dhillon, Raji _____

Dr. Diver, Skye _____

Dr. Virdee, Sumen _____

Dr. Chana, Chris _____

Dr. Climber, Rok _____

Dr. Perez, Christine _____

Dr. McDonald, Rachel _____

Dr. Racer, Car _____

Dr. Radia, Kal DDS _____

EXERCISE 2

Decide whether each of the following DEA numbers is valid or invalid. If it is invalid, explain why.

    1. AD4589624   **Valid**   **Invalid**

Explain: _____

_____

_____

    2. BD1259637   **Valid**   **Invalid**

Explain: _____

_____

_____

    3. AY8529630   **Valid**   **Invalid**

Explain: _____

_____

_____

    4. BR1235868   **Valid**   **Invalid**

Explain: _____

_____

_____

    5. A51235984   **Valid**   **Invalid**

Explain: _____

_____

_____

    6. BV1258749   **Valid**   **Invalid**

Explain: _____

_____

_____

7. BB1245786   **Valid**   **Invalid**

Explain: _____

_____

_____

8. AA7755690   **Valid**   **Invalid**

Explain: _____

_____

_____

9. AF4125736   **Valid**   **Invalid**

Explain: _____

_____

_____

10. BC1247859   **Valid**   **Invalid**

Explain: _____

_____

_____

11. AE7458963   **Valid**   **Invalid**

Explain: _____

_____

_____

12. BO4585963   **Valid**   **Invalid**

Explain: _____

_____

_____

Name_____

Lab 5: Sig Codes and Medical Terminology

OBJECTIVE ───────────────────────────────────────

By completing this exercise, the student will learn the various codes used in the pharmacy on a daily basis.

EXERCISE 1 ───────────────────────────────────────

Convert the following Sig Codes into layman's terms.

D/C _____

aa _____

bid _____

d _____

ss _____

pc _____

q _____

wa _____

atc _____

aq _____

npo _____

rep _____

mr _____

gtts _____

inj _____

opth _____

am _____

pm _____

h _____

i _____

ii _____

iii _____

iv _____

v _____

x _____

c _____

a _____

ad _____

as _____

id _____

im _____

iv _____

ivpb _____

od _____

os _____

ou _____

pr _____

pv _____

sl _____

sc _____

top _____

vag _____

nas _____

ac _____

prn _____

hs _____

stat _____

qd _____

qod _____

tid _____

qid _____

qh _____

q2h _____

q4h _____

q6h _____

q8h _____

q10h _____

q12h _____

apap _____

asa _____

bp _____

bm _____

cap _____

tab _____

liq _____

tsp _____

tbsp _____

oz _____

g _____

mg _____

po _____

mcg _____

kg _____

L _____

d5w _____

ns _____

sig _____

dx _____

mom _____

mvi _____

ha _____

n/v/d _____

NTG _____

ung _____

NKDA _____

SOB _____

tac _____

TPN _____

UTI _____

DSS _____

PCN _____

NPO _____

TCN _____

T#3 _____

T#2 _____

Sol _____

Cbc _____

UD _____

ASAP _____

MR × 1 _____

↑ incr _____

NPO _____

OTC _____

Cod _____

PRNP _____

Cre_____

HIV _____

EXERCISE 2 ──

Translate the following prescriptions.

1 tab po q 4hr prn n/v/d

_____

_____

ii tsp po prn ha atc

_____

_____

1oz q4hr pr prn n

_____

_____

1 puff q6hr prn SOB

_____

_____

1 tab prior to activity

_____

_____

Insert 1 tab po q6hr prn UTI

_____

_____

ii bid

_____

_____

iv bid

_____

_____

v tid

_____

_____

ii bid prn

_____

_____

v caps prn

_____

_____

TBSP prn

_____

_____

prn HA

_____

_____

I.V. Push

_____

_____

ii q am

_____

_____

v prn n/v

_____

_____

ii c food

_____

_____

v caps qd

_____

_____

iii fl prn qd

_____

_____

ii tabs q pm

_____

_____

iiv q hs

_____

_____

1 tsp bid-tid

_____

_____

2 tabs q 4 hrs

_____

_____

1 tab STAT

_____

_____

500mg po qid

_____

_____

1g IV prn

_____

_____

1 gtt ou bid prn

_____

_____

5ml q 8 hrs

_____

_____

4gtt AU prn p

_____

_____

15mg high BP

_____

_____

1 supp PR

_____

_____

1 gtt into AST eye

_____

_____

V gtts AD for infection

_____

_____

1 tab prn GI pain

_____

_____

od prn

_____

_____

2 tabs po q 4–5 hrs prn pain

_____

_____

ii gtts into OD prn infection × 7d, if not relief after 7d, MR × 1 for additional 7d

_____

_____

Rf 4

_____

_____

Xmls po prn

_____

_____

Apply sparingly para scalp line

_____

_____

XXX u prn insulin >6.4

_____

_____

V tabs po qid × 5d, then iv tabs po qid × 4d, then iii tabs po qid × 3d, then ii tabs qid × 2 days, then 1/2 tab qid × 1 day. Then stop

_____

_____

ii tabs po q 12 hrs for 5d, iii tabs po q8 hrs × 6d, iv tabs po q 4 hrs × 6d, 1 po TBSP bid × 4d, 1fl po qid × 4d.

_____

_____

V mls po q 12 hrs prn HA

_____

_____

1/2 tab po prior to appt

_____

_____

350L po prn electrolyte deficiency

_____

_____

ii supp vag prn infection

_____

_____

Sc, SQ sq

_____

_____

Top

_____

_____

11 tabs ATC prn N/V

_____

_____

1L prior to colonoscopy

_____

_____

v gtt AU bid × 4d, iv gtt AU bid × 4d, iii gtt AU bid × 3d.

_____

_____

3 gtts AS

_____

_____

EXERCISE 3

What do the following root words, prefixes, and suffixes mean?

Root Words

1. adeno

_____

_____

2. bucc

_____

_____

3. cardi

_____

_____

4. dermat

_____

_____

5. encephal

_____

_____

6. gastr

_____

_____

7. hemo

_____

_____

8. hepat

_____

_____

9. lacto

_____

_____

10. leuko

_____

_____

11. mal

_____

_____

12. necro

_____

_____

13. onc

_____

_____

14. oste

_____

_____

15. phleb

_____

_____

16. ren

_____

_____

17. thrombo

_____

_____

Prefixes

1. a

_____

_____

2. brady

_____

_____

3. circum

_____

_____

4. dys

_____

_____

5. ecto

_____

_____

6. endo

_____

_____

7. hyper

_____

_____

8. hypo

_____

_____

9. infra

_____

_____

10. meta

_____

_____

11. micro

_____

_____

12. neo

_____

_____

13. para

_____

_____

14. peri

_____

_____

15. poly

_____

_____

16. post

_____

_____

17. pre

_____

_____

18. retro

_____

_____

19. sub

_____

_____

20. supra

_____

_____

21. syn

_____

_____

22. tachy

_____

_____

23. trans

_____

_____

24. ultra

_____

_____

Suffixes

1. algia

_____

_____

2. cyte

_____

_____

3. dipsia

_____

_____

4. ectomy

_____

_____

5. emia

_____

_____

6. gram

_____

_____

7. itis

_____

_____

8. lepsy

_____

_____

9. malacia

_____

_____

10. megaly

_____

_____

11. osis

_____

_____

12. penia

_____

_____

13. phobia

_____

_____

14. plasty

_____

_____

15. rrhea

_____

_____

16. rrhage

_____

_____

17. sclerosis

_____

_____

18. stasis

_____

_____

19. stenosis

_____

_____

20. scopy

_____

_____

21. therapy

_____

_____

22. tomy

_____

_____

23. trophy

_____

_____

24. uria

_____

_____

Lab 6: Patient Profile

OBJECTIVE

By completing this exercise, the student will learn to calculate estimated days supply, learn to do early refills calculations, and understand what a basic patient profile may contain.

INSTRUCTIONS

Create a patient profile using the attached prescriptions. Use the provided example as a guideline and provide an estimated days supply (EDS). Remember, the insurance company will only allow a 30-day supply for all orders; the refills remaining must be adjusted accordingly. Additional patient profiles can be found in the Appendix.

Example:

Uri Spaz has been prescribed two medications:

Lipitor 40mg, 1qd #30

Naproxen 250mg, 1bid #60

Prescription 1:

Lipitor 40mg: EDS 30 days

Spaz filled his medication on 3/2/05 for a 30-day supply. Spaz may pick up his medications every 24 days. The next earliest refill date will be 4/24/08.

Prescription 2:

Naproxen 250mg: EDS: 30 days

Spaz filled the prescription on 1/8/2008. This patient has to wait until 80% of the medication is finished. Spaz may have filled the prescription on 1/31/08.

Dr. Phull, H	Dr. Diver, Skye	Dr. Bansal, S	Dr. Perez, C
Dr. Mundian, K	Dr. Virdee, S	Dr. Climber, R	Dr. Racer, C
Dr. Dhillon, S	Dr. Chana, C	Dr. McDonald, R	Dr. Radia, K

Bansal Urgent Care

Name: _Spaz, Uri_   Date: _Sample_
Address: _____
RX

  Naproxen 250mg #60
      T bid

DAW ☐   Refill ②   MD _Bansal_   Lic. No :
                      DEA#

Adventure Pharmacy

Patient Name	Uri Spaz AKA:				Sex: M / F		
Patient Address	9832 Sample Lane, CA 94560				Allergies: No Known Drug Allergies		
Patient DOB	6/9/75 Note:				Telephone # 510-862-8946		
Insurance Name	Bansal Insurance Group: 12345 Relation: Self				ID # Sandeep		
Date	Name, Strength of Medication	Directions	QTY	DS	Physician	Refills Remaining
1/8/2008	Naproxen 250mg	Take 1 tablet twice daily	60	30	Bansal, S	2
1/31/2008	Naproxen 250mg	Take 1 tablet twice daily	60	30	Bansal, S	1
3/2/2008	Lipitor 40mg	Take 1 tablet everyday	60	30	Bansal, S	3
3/5/2008	Naproxen 250mg	Take 1 tablet twice daily	60	30	Bansal, S	0
3/25/2008	Lipitor 40mg	Take 1 tablet everyday	60	30	Bansal, S	2
4/24/2008	Lipitor 40mg	Take 1 tablet everyday	60	30	Bansal, S	1
5/24/2008	Lipitor 40mg	Take 1 tablet everyday	60	30	Bansal, S	0

QTY: Quantity to be Dispensed   EDS: Estimated Day Supply

Patient 1: Irma Bullock

2834 Country Rd,
Country City, GA
   32813
    #415-555-3815

DOB: 2/17/65 (F)
Allergic: Tetracycline
    pick up 1½hrs

INS: RED POCKER
    Self
    J BRO. HILLS
    ID. ATV

Dr. Phull, H	Dr. Diver, Skye	Dr. Bansal, S	Dr. Perez, C
Dr. Mundian, K	Dr. Virdee, S	Dr. Climber, R	Dr. Racer, C
Dr. Dhillon, S	Dr. Chana, C	Dr. McDonald, R	Dr. Radia, K

Bansal Urgent Care

Name: Irma Bullock   Date: 6-9-02
Address:
RX

    Allegra 60mg #30
     Tqam

DAW ☐   Refill ④   MD Phull, H.   Lic. No :
                              DEA#

Dr. Phull, H	Dr. Diver, Skye	Dr. Bansal, S	Dr. Perez, C
Dr. Mundian, K	Dr. Virdee, S	Dr. Climber, R	Dr. Racer, C
Dr. Dhillon, S	Dr. Chana, C	Dr. McDonald, R	Dr. Radia, K

Bansal Urgent Care

Name: Irma Bullock   Date: 3-3-08
Address:
RX

    Motrin 200mg #60
     T-TT q 4-6hrs prn pain

DAW ☐   Refill ①   MD Dhillon, S.   Lic. No :
                              DEA#

Dr. Phull, H	Dr. Diver, Skye	Dr. Bansal, S	Dr. Perez, C
Dr. Mundian, K	Dr. Virdee, S	Dr. Climber, R	Dr. Racer, C
Dr. Dhillon, S	Dr. Chana, C	Dr. McDonald, R	Dr. Radia, K

Bansal Urgent Care

Name: Irma Bullock   Date: 9-3-03
Address:
RX

    Apri #1 pack
     Tqd as directed

DAW ☐   Refill ③   MD Perez, C.   Lic. No :
                              DEA#

Dr. Phull, H	Dr. Diver, Skye	Dr. Bansal, S	Dr. Perez, C
Dr. Mundian, K	Dr. Virdee, S	Dr. Climber, R	Dr. Racer, C
Dr. Dhillon, S	Dr. Chana, C	Dr. McDonald, R	Dr. Radia, K

Bansal Urgent Care

Name: Irma Bullock   Date: 5-6-07
Address:
RX

    Glyburide 5mg #60 ⑧
     Tqd

DAW ☐   Refill ③   MD Mundian, K.   Lic. No :
                              DEA#

Dr. Phull, H	Dr. Diver, Skye	Dr. Bansal, S	Dr. Perez, C
Dr. Mundian, K	Dr. Virdee, S	Dr. Climber, R	Dr. Racer, C
Dr. Dhillon, S	Dr. Chana, C	Dr. McDonald, R	Dr. Radia, K

Bansal Urgent Care

Name: Irma Bullock   Date: 3-2-08
Address:
RX

Ambien 10mg   #100
T qhs

DAW ☐   Refill (12)   MD Racer, C   Lic. No :
DEA#

Dr. Phull, H	Dr. Diver, Skye	Dr. Bansal, S	Dr. Perez, C
Dr. Mundian, K	Dr. Virdee, S	Dr. Climber, R	Dr. Racer, C
Dr. Dhillon, S	Dr. Chana, C	Dr. McDonald, R	Dr. Radia, K

Bansal Urgent Care

Name: Irma Bullock   Date: 5-3-08
Address:
RX

Diazepam 10mg #30
T qhs pm anxiety

DAW ☐   Refill (3)   MD Radia, K   Lic. No :
DEA#

Dr. Phull, H	Dr. Diver, Skye	Dr. Bansal, S	Dr. Perez, C
Dr. Mundian, K	Dr. Virdee, S	Dr. Climber, R	Dr. Racer, C
Dr. Dhillon, S	Dr. Chana, C	Dr. McDonald, R	Dr. Radia, K

Bansal Urgent Care

Name: Bullock, Irma   Date: 11-1-03
Address:
RX

Minocycline 100mg   #30
T qam x 10d

DAW ☐   Refill (2)   MD Diver, Skye   Lic. No :
DEA#

Dr. Phull, H	Dr. Diver, Skye	Dr. Bansal, S	Dr. Perez, C
Dr. Mundian, K	Dr. Virdee, S	Dr. Climber, R	Dr. Racer, C
Dr. Dhillon, S	Dr. Chana, C	Dr. McDonald, R	Dr. Radia, K

Bansal Urgent Care

Name: Bullock, Irma   Date: 1-3-03
Address:
RX

Lipitor 40mg #30
T qd

DAW ☐   Refill (4)   MD Chana, cha.   Lic. No :
DEA#

```
Dr. Phull, H        Dr. Diver, Skye     Dr. Bansal, S       Dr. Perez, C
Dr. Mundian, K      Dr. Virdee, S       Dr. Climber, R      Dr. Racer, C
Dr. Dhillon, S      Dr. Chana, C        Dr. McDonald, R     Dr. Radia, K
```

Bansal Urgent Care

Name: _Irma Bullock_   Date: _9-14-03_
Address: _____
RX

  Motrin 600mg #30
  ī-īī q4-6 hrs prn pain

DAW [X]   Refill ④   MD _Radia_   Lic. No : _____
                      DEA#

```
Dr. Phull, H        Dr. Diver, Skye     Dr. Bansal, S       Dr. Perez, C
Dr. Mundian, K      Dr. Virdee, S       Dr. Climber, R      Dr. Racer, C
Dr. Dhillon, S      Dr. Chana, C        Dr. McDonald, R     Dr. Radia, K
```

Bansal Urgent Care

Name: _Irma Bullock_   Date: _8-15-03_
Address: _____
RX

  Naprosyn 500mg #30
  ī-īī q 8 hrs prn

DAW [ ]   Refill ②   MD _Radia_   Lic. No : _____
                      DEA#

Adventure Pharmacy

Patient Name	AKA:		Sex: M / F		
Patient Address			Allergies:		
Patient DOB	Note:		Telephone #		
Insurance Name	Group:	Relation:	ID #		
Date	Name, Strength of Medication	Directions	QTY DS	Physician	Refills Remaining

QTY: Quantity to be Dispensed   EDS: Estimated Day Supply

Patient 2: Mark Damion

3158 Memory Lane
Retired City, AZ
82815

DOB: 10/16/50
allergies: Sulfa
pick up: tomorrow   spouse

#405-555-1528

INS:
Yellow Bird
ID: Damion
Group N/A

Dr. Phull, H	Dr. Diver, Skye	Dr. Bansal, S	Dr. Perez, C
Dr. Mundian, K	Dr. Virdee, S	Dr. Climber, R	Dr. Racer, C
Dr. Dhillon, S	Dr. Chana, C	Dr. McDonald, R	Dr. Radia, K

Bansal Urgent Care

Name: Mark Damion   Date: 7-7-07
Address:
RX

Bactrim DS   #14
ī bid x 7d

DAW ☐   Refill ⓪   MD Mundian, K.   Lic. No:
DEA#

Dr. Phull, H	Dr. Diver, Skye	Dr. Bansal, S	Dr. Perez, C
Dr. Mundian, K	Dr. Virdee, S	Dr. Climber, R	Dr. Racer, C
Dr. Dhillon, S	Dr. Chana, C	Dr. McDonald, R	Dr. Radia, K

Bansal Urgent Care

Name: Damion, Mark   Date: 8/8/07
Address:
RX

Prozac 70mg   #180
ī qam

DAW ☐   Refill ③   MD Climber, R.   Lic. No:
DEA#

Dr. Phull, H	Dr. Diver, Skye	Dr. Bansal, S	Dr. Perez, C
Dr. Mundian, K	Dr. Virdee, S	Dr. Climber, R	Dr. Racer, C
Dr. Dhillon, S	Dr. Chana, C	Dr. McDonald, R	Dr. Radia, K

Bansal Urgent Care

Name: Damion, Mark   Date: 5-9-05
Address:
RX

Viagra 100mg   #10
ī prior to sexual activity

DAW ☐   Refill ③   MD Racer, C   Lic. No:
DEA#

Dr. Phull, H	Dr. Diver, Skye	Dr. Bansal, S	Dr. Perez, C
Dr. Mundian, K	Dr. Virdee, S	Dr. Climber, R	Dr. Racer, C
Dr. Dhillon, S	Dr. Chana, C	Dr. McDonald, R	Dr. Radia, K

Bansal Urgent Care

Name: Mark Damion   Date: 5-9-05
Address:
RX

Alprazolam 5mg   #60
ī qd

DAW ☐   Refill ②   MD Diver, Skye   Lic. No:
DEA#

Dr. Phull, H	Dr. Diver, Skye	Dr. Bansal, S	Dr. Perez, C
Dr. Mundian, K	Dr. Virdee, S	Dr. Climber, R	Dr. Racer, C
Dr. Dhillon, S	Dr. Chana, C	Dr. McDonald, R	Dr. Radia, K

Bansal Urgent Care

Name: Mark Damion   Date: 6-9-05
Address:
RX

Xanax 5mg   #60
T qd

DAW ☐   Refill ④   MD S Bansal   Lic. No:
                        DEA#

Dr. Phull, H	Dr. Diver, Skye	Dr. Bansal, S	Dr. Perez, C
Dr. Mundian, K	Dr. Virdee, S	Dr. Climber, R	Dr. Racer, C
Dr. Dhillon, S	Dr. Chana, C	Dr. McDonald, R	Dr. Radia, K

Bansal Urgent Care

Name: Damion, Mark   Date: 4-5-07
Address:
RX

Plavix 300mg   #60
T qam

DAW ☐   Refill ③   MD S. Dhillon   Lic. No:
                        DEA#

Dr. Phull, H	Dr. Diver, Skye	Dr. Bansal, S	Dr. Perez, C
Dr. Mundian, K	Dr. Virdee, S	Dr. Climber, R	Dr. Racer, C
Dr. Dhillon, S	Dr. Chana, C	Dr. McDonald, R	Dr. Radia, K

Bansal Urgent Care

Name: Mark Damion   Date: 5-10-07
Address:
RX

ASA 81mg #60
T qam

DAW ☐   Refill ⑫   MD H Phull   Lic. No:
                        DEA#

Dr. Phull, H	Dr. Diver, Skye	Dr. Bansal, S	Dr. Perez, C
Dr. Mundian, K	Dr. Virdee, S	Dr. Climber, R	Dr. Racer, C
Dr. Dhillon, S	Dr. Chana, C	Dr. McDonald, R	Dr. Radia, K

Bansal Urgent Care

Name: Mark Damion   Date: 2-7-07
Address:
RX

NTG Patch Y400   #30
apply one patch qpm

DAW ☐   Refill ④   MD McDonald, R.   Lic. No:
                        DEA#

Dr. Phull, H	Dr. Diver, Skye	Dr. Bansal, S	Dr. Perez, C
Dr. Mundian, K	Dr. Virdee, S	Dr. Climber, R	Dr. Racer, C
Dr. Dhillon, S	Dr. Chana, C	Dr. McDonald, R	Dr. Radia, K

Bansal Urgent Care

Name: Mark Damion   Date: 10-28-06
Address: _____
RX

Motrin 400 mg #25
ꞮꞮ q 4 hrs prn severe pain

DAW ☐   Refill ②   MD Chana   Lic. No :
DEA#

Dr. Phull, H	Dr. Diver, Skye	Dr. Bansal, S	Dr. Perez, C
Dr. Mundian, K	Dr. Virdee, S	Dr. Climber, R	Dr. Racer, C
Dr. Dhillon, S	Dr. Chana, C	Dr. McDonald, R	Dr. Radia, K

Bansal Urgent Care

Name: Mark Damion   Date: 12-1-06
Address: _____
RX

Amidrine Caps
ꞮꞮ @ onset of HA, then Ɪ prn
NTE 5 caps/24 hrs

DAW ☐   Refill ①   MD Bansal   Lic. No :
DEA#

Adventure Pharmacy

Patient Name	AKA:		Sex: M / F		
Patient Address			Allergies:		
Patient DOB	Note:		Telephone #		
Insurance Name	Group: Relation:		ID #		
Date	Name, Strength of Medication	Directions	QTY DS	Physician	Refills Remaining
			QTY: Quantity to be Dispensed EDS: Estimated Day Supply		

Patient 3: Jack Splash

1134 Young St. allergies: ⇒ PCN
Surf City, CA 82821 ^"Brands Only"

INS: Blue Rock
Ⓜ ID: Diamond
Ⓜ GRP: 010
DOB: 6/9/85 ↓

Dependent + Child (only child)

#215-555-1398

Dr. Phull, H	Dr. Diver, Skye	Dr. Bansal, S	Dr. Perez, C
Dr. Mundian, K	Dr. Virdee, S	Dr. Climber, R	Dr. Racer, C
Dr. Dhillon, S	Dr. Chana, C	Dr. McDonald, R	Dr. Radia, K

Bansal Urgent Care

Name: Jack Splash Date: 2-28-06
Address:
RX

Trazodone 150mg #180
Tqpm

DAW ☒ Refill ____ MD SBansal Lic. No :
DEA#

Dr. Phull, H	Dr. Diver, Skye	Dr. Bansal, S	Dr. Perez, C
Dr. Mundian, K	Dr. Virdee, S	Dr. Climber, R	Dr. Racer, C
Dr. Dhillon, S	Dr. Chana, C	Dr. McDonald, R	Dr. Radia, K

Bansal Urgent Care

Name: Jack Splash Date: 8-8-07
Address:
RX

Diazepam 5mg #180
T bid

DAW ☐ Refill ③ MD SBansal Lic. No :
DEA#

Dr. Phull, H	Dr. Diver, Skye	Dr. Bansal, S	Dr. Perez, C
Dr. Mundian, K	Dr. Virdee, S	Dr. Climber, R	Dr. Racer, C
Dr. Dhillon, S	Dr. Chana, C	Dr. McDonald, R	Dr. Radia, K

Bansal Urgent Care

Name: Jack Splash Date: 3/2/08
Address:
RX

Prinivil 30mg #30
T qam

DAW ☐ Refill ____ MD SBansal Lic. No :
DEA#

Dr. Phull, H	Dr. Diver, Skye	Dr. Bansal, S	Dr. Perez, C
Dr. Mundian, K	Dr. Virdee, S	Dr. Climber, R	Dr. Racer, C
Dr. Dhillon, S	Dr. Chana, C	Dr. McDonald, R	Dr. Radia, K

Bansal Urgent Care

Name: Jack Splash Date: 2/28/06
Address:
RX

Viagra 100mg #6
Thr prior to sexual activity

DAW ☒ Refill ③ MD Radia. K. Lic. No :
DEA#

Dr. Phull, H	Dr. Diver, Skye	Dr. Bansal, S	Dr. Perez, C
Dr. Mundian, K	Dr. Virdee, S	Dr. Climber, R	Dr. Racer, C
Dr. Dhillon, S	Dr. Chana, C	Dr. McDonald, R	Dr. Radia, K

Bansal Urgent Care

Name: *Jack Splash* Date: 3/9/05

Address: _____

RX

Amoxil 250mg/5ml
Ʇ tsp qid × 10

DAW ☐ Refill _____ MD *Virdee S* Lic. No : _____
DEA# _____

Dr. Phull, H	Dr. Diver, Skye	Dr. Bansal, S	Dr. Perez, C
Dr. Mundian, K	Dr. Virdee, S	Dr. Climber, R	Dr. Racer, C
Dr. Dhillon, S	Dr. Chana, C	Dr. McDonald, R	Dr. Radia, K

Bansal Urgent Care

Name: *Jack Splash* Date: 9-8-07

Address: _____

RX

Valium 5mg #60
Ʇ bid

DAW ☐ Refill ② MD *Chana, Chris* Lic. No : _____
DEA# _____

Adventure Pharmacy

Patient Name	AKA:		Sex: M / F		
Patient Address			Allergies:		
Patient DOB	Note:		Telephone #		
Insurance Name	Group: Relation:		ID #		
Date	Name, Strength of Medication	Directions	QTY DS	Physician	Refills Remaining
		QTY: Quantity to be Dispensed EDS: Estimated Day Supply			

Patient 4: Chris Chickpea

Pick up in 2hrs 3215 Follow Me ave Florest City, CA 23189 #915-555-5555

Male DOB: 1/22/74 Generic OK

Dr. Phull, H	Dr. Diver, Skye	Dr. Bansal, S	Dr. Perez, C
Dr. Mundian, K	Dr. Virdee, S	Dr. Climber, R	Dr. Racer, C
Dr. Dhillon, S	Dr. Chana, C	Dr. McDonald, R	Dr. Radia, K

NKDA
NO INS

Bansal Urgent Care

Name: Chris chickpea   Date: 10-10-04
Address: _____
RX

Actos   5mg   #30
↑ qd

DAW ☐   Refill ③   MD McDonald, R   Lic. No :
DEA# _____

Dr. Phull, H	Dr. Diver, Skye	Dr. Bansal, S	Dr. Perez, C
Dr. Mundian, K	Dr. Virdee, S	Dr. Climber, R	Dr. Racer, C
Dr. Dhillon, S	Dr. Chana, C	Dr. McDonald, R	Dr. Radia, K

Bansal Urgent Care

Name: Chris Chickpea   Date: 9-10-05
Address: _____
RX

Necon 1/35   #3pck
↑ qd as directed

DAW ☒   Refill ⑫   MD Bansal, S   Lic. No :
DEA# _____

Dr. Phull, H	Dr. Diver, Skye	Dr. Bansal, S	Dr. Perez, C
Dr. Mundian, K	Dr. Virdee, S	Dr. Climber, R	Dr. Racer, C
Dr. Dhillon, S	Dr. Chana, C	Dr. McDonald, R	Dr. Radia, K

Bansal Urgent Care

Name: Chris Chickpea   Date: 7-7-02
Address: _____
RX

Cleocin T #500mls
apply sparingly to face ↑ PM.

DAW ☐   Refill ③   MD Chana, C   Lic. No :
DEA# _____

Dr. Phull, H	Dr. Diver, Skye	Dr. Bansal, S	Dr. Perez, C
Dr. Mundian, K	Dr. Virdee, S	Dr. Climber, R	Dr. Racer, C
Dr. Dhillon, S	Dr. Chana, C	Dr. McDonald, R	Dr. Radia, K

Bansal Urgent Care

Name: Chickpea, Chris   Date: 8-5-04
Address: _____
RX

Flonase   #1
↑-↑↑ into each nostril qid

DAW ☐   Refill ②   MD SBansal   Lic. No :
DEA# _____

Dr. Phull, H   Dr. Diver, Skye   Dr. Bansal, S   Dr. Perez, C
Dr. Mundian, K   Dr. Virdee, S   Dr. Climber, R   Dr. Racer, C
Dr. Dhillon, S   Dr. Chana, C   Dr. McDonald, R   Dr. Radia, K

Bansal Urgent Care

Name: Chickpea, Chris   Date: 8-25-05
Address:
RX

Vicoden ES #45
TT q4-6 hrs prn

DAW ☒   Refill ②   MD Phull, H.   Lic. No :
DEA#

Dr. Phull, H   Dr. Diver, Skye   Dr. Bansal, S   Dr. Perez, C
Dr. Mundian, K   Dr. Virdee, S   Dr. Climber, R   Dr. Racer, C
Dr. Dhillon, S   Dr. Chana, C   Dr. McDonald, R   Dr. Radia, K

Bansal Urgent Care

Name: Chris Chickpea   Date: 8-25-05
Address:
RX

Vioxx 12.5mg #30
T qd

DAW ☐   Refill ⑫   MD Bansal   Lic. No :
DEA#

Dr. Phull, H   Dr. Diver, Skye   Dr. Bansal, S   Dr. Perez, C
Dr. Mundian, K   Dr. Virdee, S   Dr. Climber, R   Dr. Racer, C
Dr. Dhillon, S   Dr. Chana, C   Dr. McDonald, R   Dr. Radia, K

Bansal Urgent Care

Name: Chris Chickpea   Date: 10-10-06
Address:
RX

Baclofen 10mg #30
T qhs

DAW ☐   Refill ①   MD Diver, Skye   Lic. No :
DEA#

Dr. Phull, H   Dr. Diver, Skye   Dr. Bansal, S   Dr. Perez, C
Dr. Mundian, K   Dr. Virdee, S   Dr. Climber, R   Dr. Racer, C
Dr. Dhillon, S   Dr. Chana, C   Dr. McDonald, R   Dr. Radia, K

Bansal Urgent Care

Name: Chris Chickpea   Date: 8-30-05
Address:
RX

Lortab 10/500 #30
T qd

DAW ☐   Refill ②   MD Phull, H.   Lic. No :
DEA#

Adventure Pharmacy

Patient Name	AKA:		Sex: M / F		
Patient Address			Allergies:		
Patient DOB	Note:		Telephone #		
Insurance Name	Group: Relation:		ID #		
Date	Name, Strength of Medication	Directions	QTY DS	Physician	Refills Remaining
QTY: Quantity to be Dispensed EDS: Estimated Day Supply					

Lab 7: Law

OBJECTIVE

By completing this exercise, the student will learn about important legal matters associated with the pharmacy profession.

INSTRUCTIONS

Working individually or as a group, answer each of the following questions. At the completion of the exercise each student or group must choose 2–3 legal issues to present to the class. By the end of this exercise, you'll have created a legal handbook for your reference.

1. What is a pharmacy technician?

_____

_____

_____

2. What duties can a pharmacy technician perform?

_____

_____

_____

3. What duties is a pharmacy technician not allowed to perform?

_____

_____

_____

4. Who is allowed into the pharmacy?

_____

_____

_____

5. What licensure is required for a pharmacy technician? If a change of address is needed, whom does the pharmacy technician need to notify?

_____

_____

_____

6. What is the pharmacy-to-technician ratio? Who is responsible for overseeing a pharmacy technician trainee?

_____

_____

_____

7. Can the pharmacist leave the pharmacy for breaks and meals?

_____

_____

_____

8. What job can the technicians perform when a pharmacist is not present?

_____

_____

_____

9. What job duties can a pharmacy intern perform?

_____

_____

_____

10. What are grounds for discipline for pharmacists and pharmacy technicians?

_____

_____

_____

11. What are misdemeanors, infractions, false representations of licensure, false representations as physician, and forgery disciplines?

_____

_____

_____

12. What is required on a prescription?

_____

_____

_____

13. What is a drug defined as?

_____

_____

_____

14. What are the requirements for a label?

_____

_____

_____

15. What is a dangerous drug?

_____

_____

_____

16. Who is allowed to dispense a drug?

_____

_____

_____

17. Who is allowed to counsel a patient?

_____

_____

_____

18. What is required on a controlled prescription?

_____

_____

_____

19. What is an emergency refill of a prescription without the prescriber's authorization?

_____

_____

_____

20. Who is allowed to own a pharmacy?

_____

_____

_____

21. What are the laws regarding dispensing of hypodermic needles?

_____

_____

_____

22. What are the stages of a clinical trial?

_____

_____

_____

23. What information must be included in a drug advertisement?

_____

_____

_____

24. Under what conditions can a drug be refilled without a prescription?

_____

_____

_____

25. Under what conditions may a generic substitution be allowed?

_____

_____

_____

26. What items need to be in a patient profile? List items for both inpatient and outpatient.

_____

_____

_____

27. What are the five schedules of controlled medications? What are the refill limits of each schedule?

_____

_____

_____

28. What are the security regulations of schedule drugs?

_____

_____

_____

29. What is the exception when prescribing a schedule II drug for the terminally ill?

_____

_____

_____

30. What form must be completed when a drug is lost or stolen?

_____

_____

_____

31. Who is allowed to order and sign for schedule drugs in the pharmacy?

_____

_____

_____

32. What does the FDA oversee?

_____

_____

_____

33. What is the Drug Efficacy Amendment?

_____

_____

_____

34. What is the Investigational Drug, New Drug Application?

_____

_____

_____

35. What is the Federal Hazardous Substance Act?

_____

_____

_____

36. What are tamper- and child-resistant packaging?

_____

_____

_____

37. What is the Omnibus Budget Reconciliation Act of 1990?

_____

_____

_____

38. What is the Durham–Humphrey Amendment of 1951?

_____

_____

_____

39. What is the Kefauver–Harris Amendment of 1962?

_____

_____

_____

40. What is the Drug Abuse Control Amendment of 1965?

_____

_____

_____

41. What is the Comprehensive Drug Abuse Prevention and Control Act of 1970?

_____

_____

_____

42. What are the requirements for OTC drugs according to the FDCA?

_____

_____

_____

43. What is the DEA and how is it involved in pharmacy law?

_____

_____

_____

44. What form is needed when transferring controlled substances to new ownership of a pharmacy?

_____

_____

_____

45. What form is needed to destroy controlled substances?

_____

_____

_____

46. Who is allowed to destroy pharmaceuticals and with whom do they register?

_____

_____

_____

Lab 8: HIV/AIDS

OBJECTIVE

This exercise will teach the student important information regarding HIV/AIDS disease and the drugs used to treat it.

INSTRUCTIONS

Answer the following questions about HIV/AIDS and discuss them with your class.

1. Define the following terms:

    a. Asymptomatic

_____

_____

_____

    b. Primary or acute HIV infection

_____

_____

_____

2. How does the HIV test work?

_____

_____

_____

3. How long can someone be infected with HIV before it becomes AIDS?

_____

_____

_____

4. What is the life cycle of HIV?

_____

_____

_____

5. What are the symptoms of AIDS?

_____

_____

_____

6. What are opportunistic infections?

_____

_____

_____

    a. What are bacterial infections?

_____

_____

_____

    b. What are viral infections?

_____

_____

_____

    c. What are fungal infections?

_____

_____

_____

    d. What are parasitic infections?

_____

_____

_____

    e. What are some other complications?

_____

_____

_____

7. What are the five stages of HIV/AIDS?

_____

_____

_____

8. What is a normal CD4 count?

_____

_____

_____

9. What does the CD4 count drop to when infected with HIV?

_____

_____

_____

10. CCL3L1 is the gene that does what?

_____

_____

_____

11. How can HIV be transmitted?

_____

_____

_____

12. What are the risk factors for HIV?

_____

_____

_____

13. What is a drug cocktail?

_____

_____

_____

14. What are secondary opportunistic infections?

_____

_____

_____

15. What is HAART?

_____

_____

_____

16. What are NRTIs?

_____

_____

_____

17. What are PIs?

_____

_____

_____

18. What are NNRTIs?

_____

_____

_____

19. What are NtRTIs?

_____

_____

_____

20. What are fusion inhibitors?

_____

_____

_____

21. Are there any alternative medicines available?

_____

_____

_____

22. Are there any new HIV/AIDS medications?

_____

_____

_____

23. What precautions should you take when helping an HIV/AIDS patient?

_____

_____

_____

24. What is a fixed-dose combination?

_____

_____

_____

25. What are synergistic enhancers?

_____

_____

_____

26. What are the common cocktails?

_____

_____

_____

PART 2

Complete the provided charts by researching the medications.

Table 8-1 NNRTIs

Brand Names	Generic Names	Formulation/Dosing	Side Effects	Drug Interactions

Table 8-2 Fusion Inhibitors

Brand Names	Generic Names	Formulation/Dosing	Side Effects	Drug Interactions

Table 8-3 Combination Drugs

Brand Names	Generic Names	Formulation/Dosing	Side Effects	Drug Interactions

Table 8-4 Protease Inhibitors

Brand Names	Generic Names	Formulation/Dosing	Side Effects	Drug Interactions

Table 8-5 NRTIs

Brand Names	Generic Names	Formulation/Dosing	Side Effects	Drug Interactions

Lab 9: What Would You Do?

OBJECTIVE ————————————————————————————————————

By completing this exercise, the student will be exposed to different scenarios and learn how to handle difficult situations in the pharmacy.

INSTRUCTIONS ————————————————————————————————

Individually or in groups, read the following scenarios and describe action the pharmacy technician should take in order to resolve the problem. Then, discuss your solutions with the class.

1. A patient walks into the pharmacy and he does not understand what you are saying to him. He looks at you with a blank stare. You explain that it will take at least 15 minutes to fill his prescription. He then says ok and just stands at the take-in counter. What do you do?

_____

_____

_____

_____

_____

2. It is 12:45, the Rph left for lunch at 12:30. A patient walks into the pharmacy and demands that she see the pharmacist right away. She has a complaint, but the pharmacist is at lunch. You explain to the patient that the pharmacist is at lunch and that she will return at 1:30. The patient becomes irate and demands to see the pharmacist immediately.

_____

_____

_____

_____

_____

3. Ms. Skydive walks into the pharmacy with a prescription for Valium. There is nothing wrong with the prescription, so you tell her it will be a 15 minute wait. After she walks away, the next patient has a prescription for Compazine (nausea/vomiting). This patient looks bad and is clearly not feeling very well. Will it be a 15 minute wait for this patient as well? Why or why not?

_____

_____

_____

_____

4. Mr. Jumper walks into the pharmacy with a prescription for Vicodin. He looks nervous, keeps asking you whether the prescription is ok, and wants you to fill the prescription as soon as possible. What should you be concerned about?

_____

_____

_____

_____

5. Mr. Rude comes in to pick up his prescription and has a $150 copay. He begins to yell at you, saying that his copay shouldn't be that high and that you do not know what you are doing! He wants you to fix the problem and wants his copay to be the $15 that it was before. What should you do?

_____

_____

_____

_____

6. Mrs. X calls in to the pharmacy and wants her prescriptions to be transferred to another pharmacy. Can you do that? Why or why not?

_____

_____

_____

_____

7. John is going on vacation tomorrow and he needs his prescriptions filled today. The problem is that he picked up his prescriptions only 14 days ago and has not finished three-fourths of his medications. What do you do?

_____

_____

_____

_____

8. You discover that a certain floor has ordered Demerol with no physicians' orders. Can a nurse order Demerol without a prescription? What would you do?

_____

_____

_____

_____

9. A patient brings an empty bottle into the pharmacy and says he ran out of his medication. When you look at the bottle you see it is a heart medication, and the patient has no refills left. Can you fill it for the patient?

_____

_____

_____

_____

10. Ms. Snooty walks into the pharmacy with an attitude and says her doctor called in the prescription for her about 3 hours ago. You check the computer and find nothing; you check the "problem box" (where all prescriptions are put if there are problems with them—for example if something needs to be verified and you are waiting for the MD to call back), and you find nothing. You look everywhere and find nothing. You tell her that you will call the doctors' office to make sure they called it in (they sometimes forget), but you get a voicemail and leave a message. You tell the patient you can page the doctor but do not know how long it will take for him to respond. She begins to yell and curse. What do you do?

_____

_____

_____

_____

11. How would you communicate with a patient who is hearing impaired?

_____

_____

_____

_____

_____

12. You are filling prescriptions and realize that your brother's girlfriend came to get a prescription to treat an STD. He is your brother, but you are aware of HIPAA regulations. What do you do?

_____

_____

_____

_____

_____

13. It is lunchtime and a patient walks in with an empty bottle of medication and asks if you can fill it for him. He has no refills and the Rph is at lunch. Can you fill it?

_____

_____

_____

_____

_____

14. The Rph asks you to call the doctors' office to verify the strength on a prescription, and the nurse decides to change it. Can you change it or do you have to give the prescription to the Rph?

_____

_____

_____

_____

_____

15. You receive a prescription that looks like it has been changed by the patient; do you tell the patient that the prescription looks like it has been altered?

_____

_____

_____

_____

_____

16. Dr. Bansal comes in with a prescription for herself for Allegra. Can you fill it? Why or why not?

_____

_____

_____

_____

_____

17. Do you have the right to refuse service to a patient? If so, under what circumstances?

_____

_____

_____

_____

_____

18. The pharmacist filled a prescription incorrectly and asks you not to say anything. What would you do?

_____

_____

_____

_____

_____

19. You are the technician and are left alone in the pharmacy while the Rph goes to lunch. Your friend comes by to see you, and you let her in. You are supervising her the whole time she is there. Is this acceptable?

_____

_____

_____

_____

_____

20. Your friends are addicted to pain medications and when they discover you have access to Vicodin, they ask you to provide them with some tablets. What would you do?

_____

_____

_____

_____

_____

21. Patient Jumper is on Medi-Cal. They are prescribed Cipro for a UTI. Under the Medi-Cal formulary a UTI is not a condition for which the medication is covered. Can the pharmacist change the diagnosis to something that is covered?

_____

_____

_____

_____

22. Patient Q has a prescription filled for HIV medications along with Vicodin. After pickup, the patient returns and tells you that his medication was run over by a bus. He would like to get his medications refilled; he only wants the Vicodin refilled. Should you fill it?

_____

_____

_____

_____

23. You are working with a pharmacist who is consistently making mistakes. Would you continue to fix his mistakes or speak to your supervisor about the situation?

_____

_____

_____

_____

_____

Lab 10: New Drug Process

OBJECTIVE ——

This exercise will expose the student to the broad process of a new drug from the point of view of pharmaceutical companies.

INSTRUCTIONS ——

Working in groups, create a new drug and present it to the class. One way to get started is to read packet inserts for medications that are related to the drug your group will be creating. For example, if your group is developing a cardiovascular drug, then a packet insert for Nitroglycerin would be helpful. This is an exercise that requires creativity so the sky is the limit for your imagination.

The following information must be included in your presentation:

1. Chemical composite: What chemicals make up the drug? Using the periodic table of contents, create a chemical breakdown. When reading the periodic table of contents, keep in mind that the numbers refer to the amount of atoms and protons in that particular element. You do need extensive knowledge of chemistry in order to create the chemical breakdown, but there must be access to a periodic table. Let's break down my favorite element, Gold:

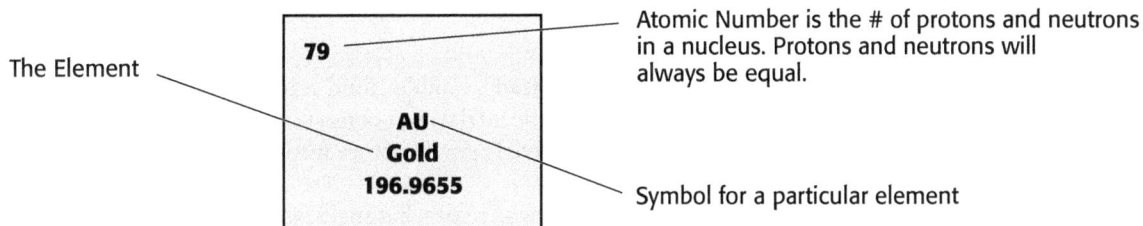

The Element

79

AU
Gold
196.9655

Atomic Number is the # of protons and neutrons in a nucleus. Protons and neutrons will always be equal.

Symbol for a particular element

For example, the following chemical description reads as follows:

HO_2: This includes 1 Hydrogen element, and 2 Oxygen elements.

C_2S_2: This includes 2 Carbon elements and 2 Sulfur elements.

FH_4: This includes 1 Fluorine element and 4 Hydrogen elements.

O_2: This includes 2 Oxygen elements.

The chemicals in my drug include Hydrogen, Oxygen, Carbon, Sulfur, and Fluorine.

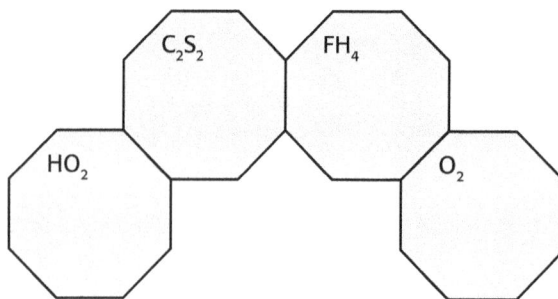

2. Method of Action (MOA): How does the chemical work in the body?

3. Food-to-Drug Interactions: Are there any types of foods that a person should stay away from while on this medication?

4. Drug-to-Drug Interactions: This occurs when two medications that interact with each other are taken together.

5. Clinical Trials: Clinical trials have four phases.

   a. Phase I: Researchers test an experimental drug or treatment in a small group of people (20–80) for the first time to evaluate its safety, determine a safe dosage range, and identify side effects.

   b. Phase II: The experimental study drug or treatment is given to a larger group of people (100–300) to see whether it is effective and to further evaluate its safety.

   c. Phase III: The experimental study drug or treatment is given to large groups of people (1,000–3,000) to confirm its effectiveness, monitor side effects, compare it to commonly used treatments, and collect information that will allow the experimental drug or treatment to be used safely.

   d. Phase IV: Postmarketing studies delineate additional information including the drug's risks, benefits, and optimal use.

There are many ways to carry out a clinical trial: blind study, double-blind study, and triple-blind study in which placebos (pills with no medication) are used. Clinical trials can consist of different age groups, specific genders, and ethnicity or race. (Please see www.clinicaltrials.gov for more information on clinical trials.)

   a. Blind Study: In a blind study the investigator is unaware of what medication the participant is being given. Having a single-blind study helps prevent bias by the investigator toward any single participant. Sometimes the participants may also be unaware of what they are being administered.

   b. Double-Blind Study: In this study neither the participant nor the investigator is aware of what medication is being administered. This type of study can be the objective.

   c. Triple-Blind Study: In this type of study those who organize the study, analyze the data, the participants, and the investigator are all unaware of the treatment.

6. Recommended Dosage: How much medication should the patient receive on a daily basis without producing a toxic effect? It is up to the group to determine the recommended dose.

7. Indications and Use: What is the medication used for? Is it for allergies, angina, pain, inflammation, etc.?

8. Contraindications: Who should not use the medications? (Pregnant women, children, men, tall people, etc.)

9. Warnings: Is there anything that might happen to the patient when they start taking this medication, such as withdrawal, immune suppression, etc.?

10. Pregnancy Category: Can pregnant women take this medication? Is it limited to a certain trimester?

11. Pediatric and Geriatric Use: Are there special considerations when administering the medication to children or the elderly?

12. Adverse Effects (Side Effects): What are the adverse effects and what percentage of the participants experienced them?

13. How Supplied: Does this come in injections, liquid, suppository, tablets, etc.?

The second half of the project includes administrative issues: The following items must be answered. Your budget consists of 5 million dollars. Remember that companies spend more on certain areas, such as advertising, than they spend on clinical trials.

1. What is the company name?

   Location?

2. Who are your sales representatives?

   What is their pay?

3. How are you advertising the medication?

   What is the cost?

4. Complete a new drug application.

   How much does this cost?

5. How much will you sell the medication for?

   What is your profit margin?

6. How much are the researchers making? (e.g., scientists, pharmacists, etc.)

7. How much are you paying clinical trial participants?

Lab 11: Sound-Alike Drugs

OBJECTIVE

This exercise will expose the student to drugs that sound alike and help them understand the consequences of mistaken medications.

INSTRUCTIONS

Sound-alike drugs are a common reason for medication errors. These drugs have either similar spelling or a similar sounding name, for example, hydralazine vs. hydroxyzine. It is easy to confuse the two medications when typing or filling a prescription. It is CRITICAL that the pharmacy technician ask the pharmacist if there is any doubt regarding a prescription.

   The following prescriptions have been prescribed to patients on the basis of their diagnosis. In each of the following cases, it is up to you to decide whether the prescription is correct. If the prescription is correct then you do not need to change anything; if it is incorrect then you must change the prescription. Answer each of the questions associated with each case.

   Using the following list of sound-alike drugs decide whether the following prescriptions are written correctly:

Retrovir, Fiorinal, Hydroxyzine, Buspirone, *Denavir, Toprol, Provera,* Ephedrine, *Xanax, Inderal, Celebrex, Nicoderm,* Sulfasalazine, *Klonopin, Ativan, Fioricet, Morphine, Oxycodone,* Hydralazine, Bupropion, Hydromorphone, *Lamictal,* Daunorubicin, Clonidine, *Retonavir, Codeine,* Lorazepam, Sulfasoxazole, Epinephrine, Nitroderm, *Covera,* Cerebyx, *Adderall, Lodiene,* Indinavir, *Lamisil*

CASE #1

Mr. Show is admitted to the hospital with an acute case of anaphylactic shock that is associated with cardiac arrest. He has already been given CPR and resuscitation attempts have failed. The doctor has administered epinephrine 0.15mg every 8 minutes to "jump start" his heart in a resuscitation effort.

   1. What, if anything, is wrong with this prescription?

_____

_____

_____

2. Are there any drug interactions?

_____

_____

_____

3. Is the correct medication prescribed for the correct indication?

_____

_____

_____

CASE #2 ——————————————————————————————————————

Mr. Dewey brings in a prescription for treatment of high blood pressure. His doctor has prescribed him hydroxyzine 25mg with directions that read 1 tablet four times a day.

1. What, if anything, is wrong with this prescription?

_____

_____

_____

2. Are there any drug interactions?

_____

_____

_____

3. Is the correct medication prescribed for the correct indication?

_____

_____

_____

CASE #3 ————————————————————————————————————

Mr. Squek brings in a prescription for treatment of his rheumatoid arthritis in his left knee. The doctor has written a prescription for cerebyx 150mg bid.

   1. What, if anything, is wrong with this prescription?

_____

_____

_____

   2. Are there any drug interactions?

_____

_____

_____

   3. Is the correct medication prescribed for the correct indication?

_____

_____

_____

CASE #4 ————————————————————————————————————

Klonopin is administered to John Doe for treatment of Lennox-Gastaut syndrome. The doctor has prescribed 0.5mg tid for 2 days. Also prescribed is clonidine for treatment of high blood pressure 0.4mg bid.

   1. What, if anything, is wrong with this prescription?

_____

_____

_____

   2. What are the warnings for the patient?

_____

_____

_____

3. Is the correct medication prescribed for the correct indication?

_____

_____

_____

CASE #5 ──

Mrs. Joseph has brought a prescription into the pharmacy for treatment of insomnia. This patient has been under stress and has been having difficulty sleeping at night. Her prescription read alprazolam 1.5mg qam and 2.5mg qhs. This patient is also taking propoxyphene.

1. What, if anything, is wrong with this prescription?

_____

_____

_____

2. Are there any drug interactions?

_____

_____

_____

3. Is the correct medication prescribed for the correct indication?

_____

_____

_____

CASE #6 ──

Mr. Case brings in a prescription for his child who is 8 years old for the treatment of partial seizures. Her doctor has written a prescription for Toprolol 25mg once a day.

1. What, if anything, is wrong with this prescription?

_____

_____

_____

2. Are there any drug interactions?

_____

_____

_____

3. Is the correct medication prescribed for the correct indication?

_____

_____

_____

CASE #7 ───────────────────────────────────

Inderal has been prescribed for the treatment as a prophylaxis of migraine occurrences. The prescription reads 200mg daily.

1. What, if anything, is wrong with this prescription?

_____

_____

_____

2. Are there any drug interactions?

_____

_____

_____

3. Is the correct medication prescribed for the correct indication?

_____

_____

_____

CASE #8

Alex Jay has a prescription written for bupropion hydrochloride to treat him for anxiety with dosage of 7.5mg twice daily for 3 days, 12.5mg for 7 days, and continuing at 17.5mg.

1. What, if anything, is wrong with this prescription?

_____

_____

_____

2. Are there any drug interactions?

_____

_____

_____

3. Is the correct medication prescribed for the correct indication?

_____

_____

_____

CASE #9

Jay is HIV positive and has been prescribed Retrovir 600mg twice daily. He has a BSA of 1.25 and has been prescribed 3.75ml of a 300mg/5ml medication.

1. What, if anything, is wrong with this prescription?

_____

_____

_____

2. Are there any drug interactions?

_____

_____

_____

3. Is the correct medication prescribed for the correct indication?

_____

_____

_____

CASE #10 ——————————————————————————————————

Student Fabio has a prescription for Provera that was written for angina after complaining of chest pain. His prescription reads 100mg three times a day.

    1. What, if anything, is wrong with this prescription?

_____

_____

_____

    2. Are there any drug interactions?

_____

_____

_____

    3. Is the correct medication prescribed for the correct indication?

_____

_____

_____

CASE #11 ——————————————————————————————————

Mrs. Galaxy has been hospitalized after a fall while rock climbing at Yosemite. She has been given an IV drop that is compounded of Lodiene for the treatment of acute pain. What medication could have been confused with Lodiene and what might the doctor have prescribed for treatment of moderate pain?

    1. What, if anything, is wrong with this prescription?

_____

_____

_____

2. Are there any drug interactions?

_____

_____

_____

3. Is the correct medication prescribed for the correct indication?

_____

_____

_____

CASE #12 ───

You receive an inpatient pharmacy technician for the day and receive a prescription for indinavir for the treatment of herpes. The prescription reads 800mg every 8 hours.

1. What, if anything, is wrong with this prescription?

_____

_____

_____

2. Are there any drug interactions?

_____

_____

_____

3. Is the correct medication prescribed for the correct indication?

_____

_____

_____

CASE #13

Mark comes in with a prescription for a migraine medication but is allergic to codeine. The doctor has prescribed him Fiorinal 1–2 capsules every 4 hours, NTE 6 capsules.

    1. What, if anything, is wrong with this prescription?

_____

_____

_____

    2. Are there any drug interactions?

_____

_____

_____

    3. Is the correct medication prescribed for the correct indication?

_____

_____

_____

CASE #14

With a bad case of toenail fungus, Ian brings in a prescription for Lamictal 300mg every day.

    1. What, if anything, is wrong with this prescription?

_____

_____

_____

    2. Are there any drug interactions?

_____

_____

_____

3. Is the correct medication prescribed for the correct indication?

_____

_____

_____

CASE #15

Smoking is a bad habit that Brandon is trying to kick. He has been prescribed Nitroderm.

1. Is the prescription correct? If not, write the correct medication.

_____

_____

_____

CASE #16

What issues could arise if the drugs sumatriptan and zolmitriptan are confused? What is each medication used for?

_____

_____

_____

CASE #17

A child is given a prescription for sulfasalazine every 8 hours for a period of 10 days. The child is still suffering from an infection 2 weeks later. Why might this child still be sick?

_____

_____

_____

CASE #18

Tiazac and Ziac are sound-alike drugs. What is the difference between the two medications?

_____

_____

_____

CASE #19

Hydromorphone is given to a child for pain after a fall off her bike. She has been hospitalized and is given her medication IM every 4–6 hours. Why can this be easily confused with morphine?

_____

_____

_____

Lab 12: 21st Century Leadership Model

Belal A. Kaifi, MPA

OBJECTIVE

As a pharmacy technician, leadership is important in the field as we move up the ladder to leadership positions. This exercise will prepare the student to become a successful leader.

Today's competitive organizations demand strategic leadership. In a pharmacy, leaders must believe in change, innovate continuously, recognize the need for challenge, and stress the importance of unity and collaboration. "In highly competitive, rapidly changing environments, caring and appreciative leaders are the ones to bet on for long-term success" (Kouzes & Posner, 2003, p. 78). The twenty-first century pharmaceutical leader must be equipped with the right tools to be effective, empathic, and efficient in all aspects of the workplace. Future pharmacy technicians will benefit by sharing insights into the following questions:

1. How can I become a more empowered leader for my success and the success of the organization?

2. How can I improve my pharmaceutical skills in the workplace?

3. How can I leverage the role of my department more strategically in the organization?

4. How can I improve my management and leadership skills to meet the needs of a changing workplace?

5. How can I foster creative thinking and innovation within the current framework of my organization?

6. How do I continue to challenge and motivate my coworkers?

The following model is a dynamic framework that will help future pharmaceutical leaders understand the importance and dynamics of organizational leadership and development. The three-step model is as follows:

1. Understand the culture.

2. Practice servant leadership.

3. Reframe the organization utilizing transformational leadership.

STEP ONE

Understanding the Culture

The first step is always to identify the organization's culture. Leadership and culture are inseparable. To really understand culture, a leader must understand the deepest level of assumptions and beliefs. An organization may have many different cultures or subcultures, or even no obvious dominant culture at the organizational level. Recognizing the cultural morale is essential to identifying and understanding the culture. Organizational cultures are created, maintained, or transformed by people. An organization's culture is, in part, also created and maintained by the organization's leadership team. Detecting and understanding the existing norms are essential before a leader can pursue change by reworking the roots of culture: "Determining what needs to be changed and articulating those changes is an essential part of the effort to manage the integration of cultural roots. If leaders want to change how the job gets done, they must understand the commitments driving the work of the program and how those commitments might need to change. Articulating those changes helps participants to see the task, the resources, and the skills they bring to the table, and the environment in which they work, differently" (Khademian, 2002, p. 64). Implementing organizational change can impact an organization's culture.

Leaders can begin by getting a clear picture of the roots of the culture, in other words, by identifying the program task, the resources, and the personnel involved in the work of the program and by understanding the environment surrounding the program (Khademian, 2002, p. 109).

A leader should first think about the primary tasks of the organization by figuring out the most efficient, effective, and productive way to complete all tasks and responsibilities. As a matter of fact, organizational culture can easily influence an organization's success; therefore, a sound leader must be able to unite, empower, and motivate all employees. The employees must understand the importance of being able to perform at a higher level because of both national and international competitors. Listening and learning to develop a sense of who the organization's competitors are can offer the leader insight into a strategic competitive advantage (Khademian, 2002, p. 114). In order to survive in this competitive society, leaders have to constantly change and implement new procedures for better and higher-quality services.

The organization's allocation of resources and its processes for evaluation and planning demonstrate its capacity to fulfill its mission, improve the quality of its performance, and respond to future challenges and opportunities. In order to get a picture of the roots of organizational culture, a leader should try to comprehend the environment within which the program operates (Khademian, 2002, p. 112). Leaders should also look for ways to broaden the base of participation. This will help the morale of the organization by encouraging teamwork and enabling an "open-door policy." Encouraging participation can be implemented by company parties, evaluations, and department meetings.

The personnel of an organization are its strongest asset. The humanistic approach to reframing organizations focuses on satisfying the needs of all employees. If employees are pleased, they will be more productive, which will result in innovation and efficiency. "Obviously the people in an organization are crucial to its performance and the quality of work life within it" (Rainey, 2003, p. 219).

The culture of an organization is the foundation of this model because the culture determines the success. "Successful companies have strong, or robust cultures committed to a deep and abiding shared purpose" (Khademian, 2002, p. 21). Once the culture of an organization has been analyzed, a leader can focus on the next step, which is being an effective servant leader.

STEP TWO

Servant Leadership Style

The second step in this model includes practicing servant leadership and ultimately gaining the trust of the employees. Some people are more naturally endowed for leadership than others. Most people can be developed into strong leaders. Servant leadership emphasizes that leaders should be attentive to the concerns of their followers and empathize with them; they should take care of them and nurture them (Northouse, 2004, p. 309). There are many different leadership styles, such as transformational, participatory, and authoritarian, which are used in organizations throughout the world.

The characteristics and benefits of a servant leader in an organization are phenomenal. A servant leader leads by pure example. As Lao-Tzu (Father of Taoism) expressed, the key qualities that great leaders possess are selflessness, unbiased leadership, acting as a midwife, and being like water (Wren, 1995, p. 70). In selflessness, the wise leader is not egocentric, which equates to being more effective and open-minded. Unbiased leadership means treating everyone equally without preconceived notions. By being a midwife, leaders do not intervene unless they absolutely have to, but would rather allow employees to work collectively to resolve dilemmas on their own. A leader is like water because a leader cleanses, purifies, and improves an organization to increase efficiency, unity, and productivity.

Being able to deliver a warm style of leadership and paying attention to everyone are key elements of gaining the trust and respect of employees. The importance of paying attention is to show people that you care, and the best way to do this is to pay attention to what they're doing, how they're feeling, who they are, and what they like and dislike. "Paying attention demands that you put others first" (Kouzes & Posner, 2003, p. 79). One should not think of paying attention as "patrolling" or "inspecting" but rather being there for all employees. "One of the most common norms appears to be that of remaining loyal to the group by sticking with the policies to which the group has already committed itself, even when those policies are obviously working out badly and have unintended consequences that disturb the conscience of each member" (Wren, 1995, p. 360).

If employees acknowledge a person as a caring and supportive leader, he or she will gain their trust, respect, and friendship. While leadership is easy to explain, it is not so easy to practice. Leadership is about behavior first and skills second. It all comes back to promoting positive expectations and having these expectations realized. A servant leader should always be in a positive mood, even though he or she may be overwhelmed with work, meetings, and interviews. A servant leader should always be willing to take a few minutes out of a busy schedule to sit down and listen to any issues an employee may have.

Servant leaders are always complimenting and motivating employees and recognizing their achievements. From this outgoing and friendly behavior, it is very easy for employees to open up and communicate how they feel about every aspect of the organization. Servant leaders will respect everyone's opinion, even if someone challenges an organizational policy. "Learning to understand and see things from another's perspective is absolutely crucial to building trusting relations and to career success" (Kouzes & Posner, 2003, p. 79). Servant leaders treat people as they would like to be treated. "You express joy in seeing others succeed, you cheer others along, and you offer supportive coaching, rather than being a militant authority figure who is out patrolling the neighborhood" (Kouzes & Posner, 2003, p. 77). The quote expresses precisely how servant leaders practice leadership.

Servant leaders are followed because people trust and respect them, rather than the skills they possess. Leadership is both similar and different from management. Management relies more on planning, organizing, and dictating skills. Leadership relies on some management skills too, but more so on qualities such as integrity, honesty, humility, courage, commitment, sincerity, passion, confidence, wisdom, determination, compassion, and sensitivity. Most people don't seek to be leaders. Those who want to be a leader can develop leadership ability. It is important to understand that "as you take the role of a caring leader; people soon begin relating to you differently" (Kouzes & Posner, 2003, p. 77). A strong leader must be able to listen, consult, involve, and explain why and how things should be done. With step one and step two in perspective, a leader can now transition into a transformational leader and reframe an organization accordingly.

STEP THREE ───

Reframing Organizations Utilizing Transformational Leadership

Once a leader has understood the culture and has gained the trust of the employees, he or she can effectively reframe and transform an organization to meet all of today's standards. "Transformational Leadership involves an exceptional form of influence that moves followers to accomplish more than what is usually expected of them. It is a process that often incorporates charismatic and visionary leadership" (Northouse, 2004, p. 169). In today's complex organizations, an effective leader must be able to assess, team-build, and motivate all of the employees. "Effective leaders help articulate a vision, set standards for performance, and create focus and direction" (Bolman & Deal, 2003, p. 340). Leadership requires life-long learning.

"Transformational leaders listen to opposing viewpoints within the organization as well as threats to the organization that may arise from outside the organizations" (Northouse, 2004, p. 182). When analyzing both organizational development methods and leadership strategies, a transformational leader must be patient, be competent, and be able to identify corporate objectives. As organizations go through organizational change on a regular basis, leaders must be able to evaluate the organization from different angles to effectively find a balance for both employees and administrators. In *Reframing Organizations*, Bolman and Deal (2003) discuss four different possible frames that can be used by leadership to assess an organization. The four frames are the structural, political, humanistic, and symbolic. Each frame encompasses different characteristics that shape an organization to act and function accordingly. Each frame has unique qualities for different settings. Certain frames can be associated to the twenty-first century style of organizational development.

The most commonly used frames in organizations are the structural and political frames. The structural frame is the most common because there is a top-down formation and one person reports to the next. The structural frame is used a lot in the military. There is a hierarchy that everyone understands and follows. This frame is very structured and does not allow much room for change or challenging authorities.

The next commonly used frame in organizations is the political frame. The political arena is complex and is described as a fierce jungle. People compete against one another for scarce resources; this competition causes confusion and chaos. The political frame forces coalitions and people start having allies and enemies, thus creating dilemmas and ineffective usage of time. Government agencies are notorious for being political arenas, in which the motto, "it's not what you know, but who you know" is very true and has been proven to be a case in point for many employees. The political frame is formed in many organizations because of the scarce resources, such as promotions, growth, incentives, and favoritism.

The humanistic frame is the newest and the most effective. The humanistic frame focuses on making the organization fit the employees' needs, because employees are an organization's primary assets. If a sound leader understands how to satisfy its employees, the organization's morale will go up and employees will be more productive, effective, and efficient, resulting in raised profits and revenues. If upper management treats employees better, they will treat their customers better, which will result in employee and customer satisfaction. Transformational leaders of the future should use this tactic to promote the humanistic element of an organization.

The symbolic frame is a new concept that has proved to help develop an organization's vision by introducing symbols to the employees to help understand the importance of the organization and what their overall mission is. Bolman and Deal (2003) discuss how Nordstrom is notorious for their outstanding customer service skills. All employees must understand the customer is always right. An example of this concept is how an older lady once returned a tire to Nordstrom; a company who does not even carry tires in their stock (Bolman & Deal, 2003, p. 245). Because of outstanding customer service, the sales counselor accepted the tire and gave the lady her money back. This Nordstrom example is symbolic and shows the importance of customer service and how organizations must be able to treat employees with dignity and respect. All employees hear this symbolic story of outstanding customer service in their orientation and understand how important customer service is and its benefits to the organization. Symbols have been proven to help organizations become more successful and goal oriented.

Some problems with the structural and political frame are that people cannot question their leaders and become accustomed to routine work. Transformational leaders should focus on theory Y rather than theory X. Theory X is when subordinates are believed by their leaders to be lazy and unproductive in organizations. Theory Y points the finger at management for not challenging the employees to become more efficient, innovative, and productive (Bolman & Deal, 2003, pp. 118–119). Also, because organizations are so structured, they cannot adapt to change, which becomes difficult in this contemporary society. When an organization is too political, time will be spent manipulating, back-biting, and arguing. This particular behavior will destroy an organization's culture and cause employees to be focused on the politics of an organization rather than its vision. In this contemporary society, there can be problems with utilizing the political and structural frame exclusively. There should be a balance of all frames and every organization should try to implement the humanistic and symbolic frames to their organizations.

The usage of multiple frames in an organization can be very beneficial in the public and private sectors because employees will finally be treated fairly. A transformational leader will have the power and ability to encourage reframing by allowing all employees to voice their opinions and focusing on a labor and management partnership. Employees will finally have a voice and will be able to work in an environment where there is a balance of different frames and not just one dominating frame that can destroy an organization. Using multiple frames to evaluate an organization will help a transformational leader understand complex issues within an organization.

As mentioned above, if employees are treated better, customers will be treated better, creating a chain reaction. Being able to analyze a problem from different perspectives and more importantly from multiple angles is the optimum strategy for transformational leaders of the future to become successful. Organizations will be more proactive and less reactive if they learn to use multiple frames. "The essence of reframing is examining the same situation from multiple vantage points. The effective transformational leader understands the importance of changing lenses regularly. Reframing offers the promise of powerful new options, but cannot guarantee a new strategy will be successful. Each frame offers distinctive advantages and each has its blind spots and shortcomings" (Bolman & Deal, 2003, p. 331).

Modern organizations need the twenty-first century model of organizational leadership and development to succeed in this highly competitive global economy. Organizations need to be reframed; leaders need characteristics such as compassion and ability to nurture; and organizational cultures must be analyzed and evaluated accordingly for optimum results. Those who want to be leaders can develop leadership ability. A strong leader must be able to listen, consult, involve, and explain why and how things should be done.

EXERCISE 1: CREATING A VISION[1]

The class should be divided into small groups. Each group is responsible for developing a vision statement for a well-known organization. The vision statement should be approximately 30 words long and should be creative and concise. Remember that a vision statement is not a general goal for the organization and should inspire the stakeholders throughout the organization. Each group should be able to justify the significance of their vision statement.

_____

_____

_____

_____

_____

EXERCISE 2: THE CHARISMATIC LEADER[1]

The class should be divided into small groups and should be given a scenario to act out. Each group should elect a leader who can motivate the employees on the basis of the circumstances outlined in each scenario.

Scenario 1: A leader needs to communicate to employees that customer service has declined, causing sales to drop 30% for two consecutive weeks. The leader should address the new vision for the company.

Scenario 2: A leader has to communicate that salaries have been frozen for another year as a result of limited business. The leader needs to motivate the employees.

Scenario 3: A leader is noticing that a customer is being mistreated by a fellow coworker. The leader needs to address the importance of respect and integrity.

Scenario 4: A leader is noticing that employees are not getting along. The leader should address the importance of teamwork and synergy.

EXERCISE 3: DEVELOPING A TEAM MISSION STATEMENT[1]

The class organizes into teams of approximately six people and appoints a team leader. The task is to develop a mission statement for a global pharmaceutical company. Remember that a mission statement contains a goal and a purpose, and it is uplifting and genuine. Allow 20 minutes for preparing the mission statement and 10 minutes for preparing a logo. The leader of each group should then be prepared to present their mission statement and logo to the class.

_____

_____

_____

_____

_____

---

[1]Adapted from: Dubrin, A.J. (2007). *Human relations: Interpersonal job-oriented skills* (9th ed). Upper Saddle River, New Jersey: Pearson Education.

EXERCISE 4: ETHICAL DILEMMAS

The class should be split up into small teams. Each team should be responsible for answering the following questions. Each team should submit their answers.

Provide an example of an action in a pharmacy that might be unethical but not illegal.

_____

_____

_____

How would you deal with a colleague in a pharmacy who treated people unfairly?

_____

_____

_____

Why is patient confidentiality important in a pharmacy?

_____

_____

_____

How can behaving ethically help a pharmacy technician provide better service?

_____

_____

_____

Give an example from the media in which a leader did something of significance that was morally right. What impact did this have on our society?

_____

_____

_____

What would you do if your coworker in a pharmacy was stealing pills for herself because she didn't have health insurance?

_____

_____

_____

EXERCISE 5: LEADERSHIP CHARACTERISTICS[2]

Place a check in the box of each of the following questions that you would answer with a "yes." If you can check more than six of these, you may be well on your way to becoming an effective leader.

	Are you willing to sacrifice your own self-interest for the good of the group?
	Do you enjoy interpreting and explaining the goals of an organization?
	Would you intervene on behalf of an employee who was being mistreated?
	Are you a team player?
	Do you inspire, energize, and motivate employees?
	Do you empower coworkers?
	Do you lead by example?
	Are you known for your integrity?
	Do you believe a proactive approach is better than a reactive approach?
	Are you assertive?
	Are you self-confident?
	Do you enjoy seeing others succeed?
	Do you believe in being accountable for your actions?

EXERCISE 6: FACT OR FICTION

Each student should decide whether the following statements are either fact or fiction and should be able to justify their responses and give examples of personal experiences.

The highest percentage of turnover occurs with new employees during the probationary period.

Fact   **Fiction**

Explain:

_____

_____

_____

---

[2]Adapted from: http://www.ianrpubs.unl.edu/epublic/live/g1481/build/g1481.pdf. Accessed May 6, 2008.

A leader has the main responsibility for introduction and orientation of new employees.

Fact   **Fiction**

Explain:

_____

_____

_____

Establishment of a respectful and positive atmosphere will make employees feel at home.

Fact   **Fiction**

Explain:

_____

_____

_____

Good habits and bad habits are developed from the very start for every employee.

Fact   **Fiction**

Explain:

_____

_____

_____

It is a good idea to ask the more responsible employees in your department to mentor the new employees.

Fact   **Fiction**

Explain:

_____

_____

_____

EXERCISE 7: ETHICAL LEADERSHIP ───────────────────────────

Pharmacy technicians are leaders who assist the pharmacist in providing optimum care for patients. As a technician, one must follow many moral obligations. Choose one of the following scenarios and write a 1 page response explaining whether you agree or disagree and why.

Scenario 1: As a technician, one always has access to the patient's profile. It is unethical for a technician to discuss any medical background of his/her patients outside the pharmacy, even if the patient is a mutual friend or family member. Technicians must maintain the highest moral and ethical conduct at all times.

Scenario 2: When doctors' offices call in to refill a prescription, it is acceptable for a technician to falsify how many times a doctor has authorized a refill on a certain medication.

Scenario 3: A pharmacist is tied up with duties and kindly asks a patient to wait. The technician feels bad for the patient and takes it upon herself to counsel the patient and give recommendations.

REFERENCES ──

Bolman, L.G., & Deal, T.E. (2003). *Reframing organizations* (3rd ed.). San Fransisco: Jossey-Bass.

Khademian, A. (2002). *Working with culture.* Washington, D.C.: CQ Press.

Kouzes, J.M., & Posner, B.Z. (2003). *Encouraging the heart.* San Francisco: Jossey-Bass.

Northouse, P.G. (2004). *Leadership theory and practice* (3rd ed.). London: Sage Publications.

Rainey, H.G. (2003). *Understanding and managing organizations* (3rd ed.). San Francisco: Jossey-Bass.

Wren, J.T. (1995). *The leader's companion: Insights on leadership through the ages.* New York: Lexington Books.

Lab 13: Drug List

OBJECTIVE

After completion of this exercise, the student will be aware of medications that are regularly prescribed in a pharmacy.

INSTRUCTIONS

Using the classroom references, complete the following table. One drug has been completed as an example.

1. Provide the alternative drug name and classification.

2. Provide the indications or use for each medication.

3. Describe the method of action.

Table 13-1 Common Medications

	Alternative Name/Classification	Indications/Use	Method of Action
Amiodarone	Cordarone/Antiarrhythmic	treat ventricular tachycardia, ventricular fibrillation	stabilize heart rhythm by affecting the electrical activity of the heart
Atacand			
Atenolol			
Avalide			
Avapro			
Benazepril			
Digoxin			
Bisoprolol/HCTZ			
Captopril			
Diovan			
Cardura			
Diltiazem SR			
Clonidine			

Enalapril			
Coreg			
Lasix			
Coumadin			
Cozaar			
Toprol XL			
Triamterene/HCTZ			
Hyzaar			
Inderal LA			
Lisinopril			
Lisinopril/HCTZ			
Lotrel			
Metoprolol			
Nitroquick			

(continues)

Table 13-1 (*continued*)

	Alternative Name/Classification	Indications/Use	Method of Action
Monopril			
Nifedipine ER			
Norvasc			
Sprionolactone			
Terazosin			
Actos			
Glipizide			
Avandia			
Amaryl			
Glyburide			
Metformin ER			
Humalog			
HCTZ			

Glyburide/Metformin			
Abilify			
Effexor XR			
Cymbalta			
Lorazepam			
Lithium Carbonate			
Doxepin			
Buspirone			
Ambien			
Alprazolam			
Citalopram			
Fluoxetine			
Clonazepam			
Bupropion SR			

(continues)

Table 13-1 (*continued*)

	Alternative Name/Classification	Indications/Use	Method of Action
Diazepam			
Amitriptyline			
Lexapro			
Seroquel			
Concerta			
Strattera			
Zyprexa			
Adderall XR			
Temazepam			
Risperdal			
Paroxetine			
Nortriptyline			
Mirtazapine			

(continues)

			Zoloft
			Trazodone
			Amoxil
			Biaxin XL
			Cefzil
			Tamiflu
			Tetracycline
			Ketek
			Cipro
			Avelox
			Cephalexin
			Azithromycin
			BenzaClin
			Cefuroxime

Table 13-1 (*continued*)

	Alternative Name/Classification	Indications/Use	Method of Action
Bactroban			
Omnicef			
Nitrofurantoin			
Minocycline			
Metronidazole			
Nystatin			
Levaquin			
Apri			
Premarin			
Estradiol			
Estrostep Fe			
Evista			
Levothroid			

(continues)

Vivelle DOT			
Necon 1/35			
Nuvaring			
Ortho Evra			
Ortho Tri-Cyclen			
Prempro			
Yasmin 28			
Crestor			
Lipitor			
Lovastatin			
Tricor			
Niaspan			
Advair Diskus			
Albuterol			

Table 13-1 (*continued*)

	Alternative Name/Classification	Indications/Use	Method of Action
Allegra			
Astelin			
Clarinex			
Combivent			
Flonase			
Hydroxyzine			
Rhinocort Aqua			
Singulair			
Zyrtec			
Benadryl			
Claritin			
Celebrex			
Diclofenac			

			Indomethacin
			Etodolac
			Motrin
			Methocarbamol
			Mobic
			Nabumetone
			Naproxen
			Piroxicam
			Bentropine
			Carbidopa/Levodopa
			Ditropan XL
			Dicyclomine
			Aciphex
			Acyclovir

(continues)

Table 13-1 (*continued*)

	Alternative Name/Classification	Indications/Use	Method of Action
Alphagan P			
Aricept			
Baclofen			
Benzonatate			
Carisprodol			
Clobetasol			
Depakote			
Detrol LA			
Dilantin			
Lomotil			
Flexeril			
Allopurinal			
Flomax			

Fluconazole	Omeprazole	Fosamax	Gabapentin	Gemfibrozil	Hydroxychloroquine	Imitrex	Ketoconazole	Lamictal	Lamisil	Lescol XL	Levitra	Lidoderm	Lunesta

(continues)

Table 13-1 (*continued*)

	Alternative Name/Classification	Indications/Use	Method of Action
Methyprednisolone			
Metoclopramide			
Miacalcin			
Nexium			
Plavix			
Promethazine			
Protonix			
Skelaxin			
Tamoxifin			
Topamax			
Trileptal			
Ultracet			
Valtrex			

Viagra			
Vytorin			
Xalatan			
Zetia			
Zocor			
Cocaine			
Codeine			
Dronabinol			
Fentanyl			
Flurazepam			
Ketamine			
Meperidine			
Nandrolone			
Oxazepam			

(continues)

Table 13-1 (*continued*)

Alternative Name/Classification	Indications/Use	Method of Action
Pentobarbital		
Pentazocine		
Phenobarbital		
Stanozolol		

Lab 14: Recall

OBJECTIVE

Recalls are part of the pharmacy profession, and through this exercise the student will learn the different classes of recalls and research recalled medications.

EXERCISE 1

Instructions

Define what each type of recall means. Then using the recall classes, pick two recalls from the FDA (www.FDA.gov) and explain what type of recall it falls into and why. For example, what type of recall category would Vioxx be classified as according to the FDA? Below is a recall example provided which has been obtained from the FDA.

- **Class I recall:**

_____

_____

_____

- **Class II recall:**

_____

_____

_____

- **Class III recall:**

_____

_____

_____

- **Market withdrawal:**

_____

_____

_____

- **Medical device safety alert:**

_____

_____

_____

Sample Recall from www.fda.gov

Recall—Firm Press Release

FDA posts press releases and other notices of recalls and market withdrawals from the firms involved as a service to consumers, the media, and other interested parties. FDA does not endorse either the product or the company.

Baxter to Proceed with Recall of Remaining Heparin Sodium Vial Products

Contact:
Erin Gardiner, (847) 948-4210
Deborah Spak, (847) 948-2349

FOR IMMEDIATE RELEASE—DEERFIELD, Ill., February 28, 2008—Baxter International Inc. announced today that the company is proceeding with the voluntary recall of all remaining lots and doses of its heparin sodium injection multidose, single-dose vials and HEP-LOCK heparin flush products.

The company initially recalled nine lots of heparin sodium injection multidose vials on January 17, 2008 as a precautionary measure due to a higher than usual number of reports of adverse patient reactions involving the product and suspended production earlier this month.

Given the widespread use of this blood thinner and the impact a product shortage would have on operating rooms, dialysis centers and other critical care areas, the FDA and Baxter concluded that removing additional lots and doses of Baxter's heparin from the market earlier would have created more risk to patients requiring heparin therapy than the increased potential for experiencing an adverse reaction. Accordingly, the FDA and Baxter decided not to recall all Baxter heparin vial products at that time. The FDA has now concluded that there is sufficient capacity on the part of other suppliers that Baxter's recall will not jeopardize access to this drug, and has told Baxter that the company can now proceed with recalling its remaining heparin sodium injection and heparin flush products.

Although the vast majority of the reports of adverse reactions have been associated with the multidose products, Baxter is taking the precautionary step of recalling all remaining heparin sodium injection and heparin flush products that are currently on the market. In addition to the previously recalled lots of heparin sodium injection 1000 units/mL 10mL and 30mL multidose vials, Baxter's recall will now include the remaining lots of those products and heparin sodium injection 5000 units/mL 10mL multidose vials, heparin sodium injection 10,000 units/mL 4mL multidose vials, heparin sodium injection 1000 USP units/mL, 5000 USP units/mL, and 10,000 USP units/mL single-dose vials, and all HEP-LOCK and HEP-LOCK U/P, 10 USP units/mL and 100 USP units/mL vials, both preserved and preservative-free.

This recall does not involve Baxter's heparin pre-mix IV solutions in bags: heparin sodium in 5% dextrose injection and heparin sodium in 0.9% sodium chloride injection. "We have assurance from the U.S. Food and Drug Administration that there is an adequate supply in the market to meet the demand for these critical and lifesaving drugs," said Peter J. Arduini, president of Baxter's Medication Delivery business. "The safety and quality of our products is always our highest priority, and we will continue to collaborate with the FDA as we work to determine the cause of the increased rate of adverse reactions and resolve this issue."

Nearly all reported adverse reactions have occurred in three specific areas of product use—renal dialysis, invasive cardiovascular procedures and apheresis procedures. Reported adverse patient reactions have included: stomach pain or discomfort, nausea, vomiting, diarrhea, decreased or low blood pressure, chest pain, fast heart rate, dizziness, fainting, unresponsiveness, shortness of breath, the feeling of a strong or rapid heartbeat, drug ineffectiveness, burning sensation, redness or paleness of skin, abnormal sensation of the skin, mouth or lips, flushing, increased sweating, decreased skin sensitivity, headache, feeling unwell, restlessness, watery eyes, throat swelling, thirst, bleeding tendencies and difficulty opening the mouth. Some of these reactions, particularly profound and refractory hypotension, may be severe or life-threatening.

Customers have been instructed to discontinue use and segregate the recalled product from the rest of their inventory. Customers should then contact Baxter to arrange for return and replacement product. Customers with recalled product purchased indirectly should contact their wholesaler or distributor for return and replacement product. Customers with questions may contact the Center for One Baxter at 1-800-4-BAXTER (1-800-422-9837). Representatives will be available twenty-four hours a day, seven days a week.

FDA Recall 1: _____

What type of recall it is: _____

Why? _____

_____

_____

_____

_____

FDA Recall 2: _____

What type of recall it is: _____

Why? _____

_____

_____

_____

_____

EXERCISE 2

Instructions

Using the following information, determine which MedWatch Reporting Form the individual should use and explain why. These forms can be located and downloaded at http://www.fda.gov/medwatch/. The following scenarios are all hypothetical.

1. Bobby Ray has a prescription for Express 50mg qd, written on 6/26/02. He suffers from Egoitis, which is an inflammation of his ego. The recommended dose is 25mg po bid, or 50mg po qd. The patient is 25 years old, weighs 210 lbs, and has no other medical conditions. Within a month of taking the medication, Bobby Ray

began to complain of chest pains. Other complaints included nausea, dizziness, and diarrhea. Blood tests were taken to rule out CHD or any other cardiovascular disease. Diabetes and allergies are genetic in his family history. Medication was discontinued 7/27/02. Bobby passed away on 8/02/02.

Which reporting form should be used?_____

Why?_____

_____

_____

2. Bobby Ray has a prescription for Express 50mg qd, written on 6/26/02. He suffers from Egoitis, which is an inflammation of his ego. The recommended dose is 25mg po bid, or 50mg po qd. The patient is 25 years old, weighs 210 lbs, and has no other medical conditions. Within a month of taking the medication, Bobby Ray began to complain of chest pains. Other complaints included nausea, dizziness, and diarrhea. Blood tests were taken to rule out CHD or any other cardiovascular disease. Diabetes and allergies are genetic in his family history. Medication was discontinued 7/27/02. The patient stopped taking the medication and has provided the tablets to the doctor. After a call to the pharmacy, Dr. Detail is informed that Express 50mg tablets should be yellow, but the medication Bobby was taking was marked with the numbers 25. It is concluded that the manufacturer has made a mistake in the packaging of Express.

Which reporting form should be used?_____

Why?_____

_____

_____

Name_____

Lab 15: Infectious Disease

OBJECTIVE

As a pharmacy technician, infectious diseases, such as the flu, are common. In this exercise, the student will learn about different types of diseases outside the United States as well as medication treatment and governmental policy.

INSTRUCTIONS

According to the World Health Organization (www.who.int/en/) infectious diseases are caused by pathogenic microorganisms, such as bacteria, viruses, parasites, or fungi; the diseases can be spread, directly or indirectly, from one person to another. It is your job as a researcher to put together information about a country and the rate of infection. The following questions MUST be answered.

1. What country will your group focus on? (U.S. and Britain are not allowed)

_____

2. What disease will your group focus on and why?

_____

_____

_____

3. What are the risk factors for people living in this country?

_____

_____

_____

4. What is the treatment?

_____

_____

_____

5. What are the problems that this country is facing in regards to healthcare accessibility? What needs to be done to correct the problem?

_____

_____

_____

6. What is the government doing to help prevent disease?

_____

_____

_____

7. What is the prevalence rate per 1000 people?

Prevalence is calculated with the following information:

$$\frac{\text{\# Of cases that are present in the population at a specific time} \times 1000}{\text{\# Of people in the population at a specific time}}$$

Example: If there are 5000 people living in Jumperville, and 1258 have disease X, what is the prevalence of disease X?

$$\frac{1258}{5000} \times 1000 = 251 \text{ people have the disease per 1000 people}$$

_____

_____

_____

8. What is the cause-specific mortality rate? What is the rate of death from that particular disease? Mortality rate could be used to compare diseases to one another. For example, the student can use the mortality rate for breast cancer and lung cancer to see which one has a higher mortality rate. In order to have a fair comparison, the population must be almost equal.

$$\frac{\text{\# Of deaths due to OD}}{\text{\# Of people in the population}} \times 100$$

$$\frac{50000}{150000} \times 100\% = 33\%$$

_____

_____

_____

9. What medications would you suggest be used other than those listed?

_____

_____

_____

10. Are these blood-borne pathogens?

_____

_____

_____

11. How is it transmitted?

_____

_____

_____

REFERENCES

*Prevalence rate, mortality rate, 5 year survival rate was obtained from: Gordis, Leon. (2004). Epidemiology (3rd ed.). Philadelphia, PA: W.B. Saunders Company.

Lab 16: Medicare

OBJECTIVE ——

In this lab, the student will research the different types of Medicare for their state in order to understand the different options for Medicare plans.

INSTRUCTIONS ——

What is the lower-cost generic in your state for the following prescriptions? To determine the correct answer, use the following prescriptions and write your answer on the prescriptions themselves. Each patient has more than one prescription. After listing each medication, determine the best plan for the patient.

Step 1. Go to www.medicare.gov.

Step 2. Click on the link "Formulary Finder."

Step 3. Pick your state.

Step 4. Click on the link that says "Click here to browse drugs alphabetically."

Step 5. Create a "My Drug List" for each of the following prescriptions by selecting the appropriate drug from the alphabetical list and clicking "Add Selected Drug to the List."

Step 6. Click "Continue with Selected Drugs."

Step 7. Complete the "Quantity/Days Supply" portion, then click "Continue with Selected Drugs."

      Example:

                    Singulair 10mg # 60

                    1 qd

                    Quantity = 60, and Days Supply = every two months

Step 8. What are the top two plans for this patient?

      Answer(s): _____

Dr. Phull, H	Dr. Diver, Skye	Dr. Bansal, S	Dr. Perez, C
Dr. Mundian, K	Dr. Virdee, S	Dr. Climber, R	Dr. Racer, C
Dr. Dhillon, S	Dr. Chana, C	Dr. McDonald, R	Dr. Radia, K

Bansal Urgent Care

Name: *Patient Medicare*   Date: _____
Address: _____
RX

Epoetin Alfa 2000 u
Use as directed × 30 days

DAW ☐   Refill ③   MD *Bansal*   Lic. No : _____
DEA# _____

Dr. Phull, H	Dr. Diver, Skye	Dr. Bansal, S	Dr. Perez, C
Dr. Mundian, K	Dr. Virdee, S	Dr. Climber, R	Dr. Racer, C
Dr. Dhillon, S	Dr. Chana, C	Dr. McDonald, R	Dr. Radia, K

Bansal Urgent Care

Name: *Patient medicare*   Date: _____
Address: _____
RX

Ezetimibe 10 mg #30
T qam

DAW ☐   Refill ④   MD *Racer, C.*   Lic. No : _____
DEA# _____

Dr. Phull, H	Dr. Diver, Skye	Dr. Bansal, S	Dr. Perez, C
Dr. Mundian, K	Dr. Virdee, S	Dr. Climber, R	Dr. Racer, C
Dr. Dhillon, S	Dr. Chana, C	Dr. McDonald, R	Dr. Radia, K

Bansal Urgent Care

Name: *Patient medicare*   Date: _____
Address: _____
RX

Tyco #3 #50
T-TT q 4-6hrs prn HA

DAW ☐   Refill ⓪   MD *Diver, Skye*   Lic. No : _____
DEA# _____

Dr. Phull, H	Dr. Diver, Skye	Dr. Bansal, S	Dr. Perez, C
Dr. Mundian, K	Dr. Virdee, S	Dr. Climber, R	Dr. Racer, C
Dr. Dhillon, S	Dr. Chana, C	Dr. McDonald, R	Dr. Radia, K

Bansal Urgent Care

Name: *Medicare, Patient*   Date: _____
Address: _____
RX

Bextra 20 mg #30
T qam

DAW ☐   Refill ⑤   MD *Chana, C.*   Lic. No : _____
DEA# _____

Dr. Phull, H   Dr. Diver, Skye   Dr. Bansal, S   Dr. Perez, C
Dr. Mundian, K Dr. Virdee, S   Dr. Climber, R   Dr. Racer, C
Dr. Dhillon, S Dr. Chana, C   Dr. McDonald, R Dr. Radia, K

Bansal Urgent Care

Name: Patient medicare   Date: ___
Address: ___
RX

Ability 15 mg #60
T qd

DAW ☐   Refill ③   MD Perez, C   Lic. No : ___
DEA#

Dr. Phull, H   Dr. Diver, Skye   Dr. Bansal, S   Dr. Perez, C
Dr. Mundian, K Dr. Virdee, S   Dr. Climber, R   Dr. Racer, C
Dr. Dhillon, S Dr. Chana, C   Dr. McDonald, R Dr. Radia, K

Bansal Urgent Care

Name: P. medicare   Date: ___
Address: ___
RX

Mavix 2 mg #30
T qd

DAW ☐   Refill ①   MD Perez, C.   Lic. No : ___
DEA#

Dr. Phull, H   Dr. Diver, Skye   Dr. Bansal, S   Dr. Perez, C
Dr. Mundian, K Dr. Virdee, S   Dr. Climber, R   Dr. Racer, C
Dr. Dhillon, S Dr. Chana, C   Dr. McDonald, R Dr. Radia, K

Bansal Urgent Care

Name: Medicare, Patient   Date: ___
Address: ___
RX

Paxil 20 mg #15
T qd

DAW ☐   Refill ⑤   MD Perez, C   Lic. No : ___
DEA#

Dr. Phull, H   Dr. Diver, Skye   Dr. Bansal, S   Dr. Perez, C
Dr. Mundian, K Dr. Virdee, S   Dr. Climber, R   Dr. Racer, C
Dr. Dhillon, S Dr. Chana, C   Dr. McDonald, R Dr. Radia, K

Bansal Urgent Care

Name: Patient medicare   Date: ___
Address: ___
RX

Tacrine 10 mg #120
T qid

DAW ☐   Refill ⑤   MD S Bansal   Lic. No : ___
DEA#

Dr. Phull, H	Dr. Diver, Skye	Dr. Bansal, S	Dr. Perez, C
Dr. Mundian, K	Dr. Virdee, S	Dr. Climber, R	Dr. Racer, C
Dr. Dhillon, S	Dr. Chana, C	Dr. McDonald, R	Dr. Radia, K

Bansal Urgent Care

Name: _Patient Medicare_   Date: _____
Address: _____
RX

Xanax 0.25mg #30
Tqhs prn sleep

DAW ☐   Refill ①   MD _Bansal_   Lic. No : ____
                          DEA# _____

Dr. Phull, H	Dr. Diver, Skye	Dr. Bansal, S	Dr. Perez, C
Dr. Mundian, K	Dr. Virdee, S	Dr. Climber, R	Dr. Racer, C
Dr. Dhillon, S	Dr. Chana, C	Dr. McDonald, R	Dr. Radia, K

Bansal Urgent Care

Name: _Patient Medicare_   Date: _____
Address: _____
RX

Hivid 0.750mg #90
T q8hrs

DAW ☐   Refill ③   MD _Bansal_   Lic. No : ____
                          DEA# _____

Lab 17: Drug Information Handbook

OBJECTIVE

This exercise will familiarize the student with referencing materials used in the pharmacy.

The Drug Information Handbook

Lacy, C.F., Armstrong, L.L., Goldman, M.P., Lance, L.L. (2006). *Drug Information Handbook*. Hudson, OH: Lexi-Comp.

Covers U.S.- and Canadian-approved names of generic and trade medications.

Monograph of drug products

Pediatric and adult dosing

Labeled and unlabeled

Indications

Action, dosage, and adverse effects

Dietary considerations

Pregnancy and breast-feeding implications

INSTRUCTIONS

Use the *Drug Information Handbook* to answer the questions below. When answering the questions, include the page number where you found the information.

1. Patient A has been prescribed Mefloquine as an anti-infection medication. The directions read to take 1 tablet 1 week prior to arriving on vacation, continuing weekly during travel, and then take 1 tablet weekly for 4 weeks after returning from vacation.

    a. Is the pharmacological category correct?

_____

_____

_____

    b. What is the pregnancy category?

_____

_____

_____

2. Answer the following questions regarding the medication chloroquine.

    a. What is the brand name?

_____

_____

_____

    b. What are the monitoring parameters?

_____

_____

_____

3. Famciclovir has been prescribed to a patient with the following directions: 500mg q 8 hours for 7 days.

    a. What is the diagnosis for this medication?

_____

_____

_____

    b. Are there any drug interactions with this medication?

_____

_____

_____

4. Patient B is given ibuprofen 800mg q 4 hrs. The patient has been admitted to the hospital 3 days later for renal failure. What is the cause of the renal failure?

_____

_____

_____

5. Patient C has been prescribed a hydrochlorthiazide for high blood pressure. This patient is also taking a sulfonamide drug. Within 1 day the patient has a cardiovascular adverse reaction.

    a. What could be the reason for this occurrence?

_____

_____

_____

    b. What are some drug-to-drug interactions?

_____

_____

_____

6. What is the pregnancy category and definition for Keflex?

_____

_____

_____

7. What is the dosing restriction for an adult patient who suffers from insomnia with a prescription for Lorazepam?

_____

_____

_____

8. Using the Acetaminophen Toxicity Nomogram, identify when there will be possible hepatic toxicity.

_____

_____

_____

9. How long is Iodine 125 present in the milk of breast-feeding mothers?

_____

_____

_____

10. Using the Comparative Drug Charts, identify the first line of treatment for a generalized tonic-clonic seizure.

_____

_____

_____

11. Using the Therapy Recommendations Appendix, identify the drug regimen for Helicobacter Pylori Treatment.

_____

_____

_____

12. Which medications may precipitate depression?

_____

_____

_____

13. Under the Miscellaneous section, identify the medications that cause fevers.

_____

_____

_____

14. Which medications should not be crushed?

_____

_____

_____

15. Using the Appendix for infectious disease–prophylaxis, identify the four scenarios for prevention of perinatal HIV-1 transmission.

_____

_____

_____

Lab 18: Physicians' Desk Reference

OBJECTIVE

This exercise will familiarize the student with referencing materials used in the pharmacy.

INSTRUCTIONS

As a pharmacy technician there may come a time where you will be required to perform some research for the pharmacist. Answer the following questions by using the *Physicians' Desk Reference*.[1] The *Physicians' Desk Reference* contains five sections (found in the table of contents) that are pertinent in this exercise.

- Manufacturers' Index

- Brand and Generic Name Index

- Product Category Index

- Product Identification Guide

- Product Information

SECTION 1

1. Where is the Immunex Corporation located?

_____

_____

_____

2. For direct inquiries for Glenwood, Inc., what number should you call?

_____

_____

_____

---

[1]*Physicians' Desk Reference*. (2002). Montvale, NJ: Medical Economics Company.

3. Geneva Pharmaceuticals has two names; what is the other?

_____

_____

_____

4. Where is 3M Pharmaceuticals located?

_____

_____

_____

5. Rico Pharmacal is a subsidiary of whom?

_____

_____

_____

SECTION 2 ————————————————————————————

1. How many different types of cocaine hydrochloride are available?

_____

_____

_____

2. What are three names for desonide?

_____

_____

_____

3. How many different coenzyme Q 10 products are available?

_____

_____

_____

4. Name the different heparin sodium solutions available.

_____

_____

_____

5. What is another name for phenylephrine?

_____

_____

_____

SECTION 3 ────────────────────────────────────

1. What are some categories under cardiovascular agents? How many are there in total?

_____

_____

_____

2. Famvir is classified under which category?

_____

_____

_____

3. How many groups of antiarrhythmics are there?

_____

_____

_____

4. Is shaving cream considered a category?

_____

_____

_____

5. How many subcategories are there for laxative?

_____

_____

_____

SECTION 4

1. Draw a Depakote Sprinkle.

2. Trandate is available in what strengths?

_____

_____

_____

3. Draw the Mextil capsules.

4. What is the difference in the Apresazide capsules besides their strengths?

_____

_____

_____

5. Patient Bansal gives the technician a Risperdal tablet; how do you know what strength it is?

_____

_____

_____

SECTION 5

1. How many mgs of caffeine are in the medication Esgic?

_____

_____

_____

2. Draw the chemical structure of Darvon.

3. How is Retin-A supplied?

_____

_____

_____

4. What is the microbiology in regards to Floxin?

_____

_____

_____

5. Can Robaxin Injectable be refrigerated after mixing with I.V. fluids?

_____

_____

_____

SECTION 6

1. Where is the nearest certified poison control center?

_____

_____

_____

2. What is the number to the office of orphan products development?

_____

_____

_____

Lab 19: Inpatient Pharmacy Technician

OBJECTIVE

By completing this exercise, the student will learn how to complete patient medication administration reports.

The use of pharmacy technicians first came into being in the 1960s in teaching hospitals and was tied to changes in the practice of pharmacy. With an increasing amount of drugs on the market and an increasing hospital patient population, the demand for pharmacists began to exceed the supply of pharmacists. In addition, there were new safety initiatives in hospitals to improve medication use, such as unit dose systems and clinical pharmacy programs. By creating a group of paraprofessionals who could perform some dispensing and compounding functions, pharmacists were freed up to expand into these more sophisticated areas of pharmacy practice.

The success of pharmacy technicians in the hospital setting later led to the expansion of pharmacy technicians into retail pharmacies and also to technicians' eventual licensure by the state boards of pharmacy. Technicians are generally limited by state laws that require their work to be under the supervision of pharmacists and most of their work to be checked by pharmacists.

HOSPITAL PHARMACY

Hospital pharmacies are different from retail pharmacies in both the type of work required and the degree of patient contact. There is little direct patient contact in hospital pharmacies, whereas there is a lot of patient contact in the retail setting. In addition, hospital pharmacies are more regulated by outside agencies, like the Joint Commission (which accredits hospitals) as well as by state boards of pharmacy (which regulate both retail and inpatient settings). Hospital pharmacies vary greatly in practice from one another. Most hospital pharmacies utilize the unit dose system of medication distribution. The creation of unit dose systems led to the widespread use of pharmacy technicians in the hospital setting. The unit dose system is a medication dispensing system whereby:

- the number of doses dispensed is limited (usually not more than a 24-hour supply)

- doses are dispensed in individually packaged and labeled doses (sometimes in exact amounts as per the prescription)

- technicians do the packaging, labeling, and dispensing, which is then checked by a pharmacist

- there is a three-tiered safety check system before the dose gets to the patient: the technician filling, the pharmacist (who checks the technician), and the nurse (who checks the pharmacist's dispensed doses)

Hospital pharmacies have a central pharmacy and in larger hospitals may have smaller auxiliary pharmacies called satellites. Larger hospital pharmacies are usually open 24/7; smaller hospital pharmacies that are not always open have pharmacists on call for after-hours emergencies. For pharmacies that are not always staffed, there is an emergency supply of medications available to nurses at all times.

Pharmacy Systems

In every hospital pharmacy the workflow is similar: physicians write orders, those orders are sent to the pharmacy, the orders are transcribed for pharmacy-dispensing functions, and medications are dispensed and administered to patients by nurses. Pharmacists are required in hospitals to review all medication orders, except emergency orders for which a physician is present. Pharmacies are typically divided into two sections: the compounding IV room (for injectable medications that need special compounding) and the unit dose section (for everything else, not dispensed in the IV room). Even though this workflow is universal to hospital pharmacies, there are a variety of differences in how hospitals perform these functions.

Order Entry/Transcription

Hospital pharmacies either use a paper system of order entry (with handwritten orders) or an electronic one. There are two types of electronic systems:

- **Pharmacy systems**, which are electronic and require handwritten orders to be transcribed into an electronic ordering system.

- **CPOE** (Computerized Physician Order Entry), where the physicians enter the orders directly into the computer and there is no order transcription.

CPOE is considered safer than order transcription since there is no handwriting to read (a source of errors) and there is no rewriting of the orders into a second system (another possible source of transcription errors). As many as one-third of medication errors in hospitals can be attributed to transcription errors.

In hospitals with pharmacy systems, it is common practice for technicians to enter handwritten orders into the electronic system and for these orders to then be checked by a pharmacist. Most CPOE systems also have electronic charting of medications and other medically related treatments and tests for the patient's stay in the hospital.

Patient Profiles   In hospitals, a lot of information must be gathered on patients to help in properly prescribing drugs. These elements include name, diagnosis, primary physician, allergies, age, height, weight, and unique identification numbers assigned to patients to identify them and to help prevent errors (since there can be patients with the same or similar names in the hospital at the same time).

In addition, a properly composed order must always include:

- Drug name (what)

- Dose (how much)

- Route of administration (how and where to give)

- Frequency (how often to give)

Once a properly composed order is received on a particular patient, the order is transcribed into a dispensing record (patient profile), the order is reviewed for appropriateness and correctness by the pharmacist and then the order is set up to dispense. The patient profile is a record of all the information needed for drug dispensing and serves as the method of dispensing for cart fills and reorders. The profile shows all the current orders and also the orders that have been discontinued. Drugs can be dispensed in the maximum amount ordered by the physician (i.e., four tablets if the drug is ordered four times a day). To prevent medication errors, the exact amount must be dispensed for scheduled medications. In addition, controlled substances are never dispensed with noncontrolled medications.

Controlled Substances   Controlled substances are medications for which there is potential for abuse (such as narcotics or sleeping pills). They are classified by the DEA as Schedules I-V, with Schedule I having the highest abuse potential and Schedule V the lowest abuse potential. Controlled substances can only be handled by licensed personnel (usually doctors, nurses, and pharmacy staff) and are locked up both in the pharmacy and on the nursing units. Each dose, or partial dose, must be accounted for and careful records are maintained of all uses of controlled substances. Controlled substances are noted on patient profiles, but are not dispensed from the profile.

Dispensing

Hospital pharmacies dispense medication in a number of ways.

New orders are dispensed for a set period of time (usually for 24 hours but it may be more or less) along with dispensing for the initial order transcription.

Standing orders (orders that are still valid longer than the time period for which the initial doses are sent) are filled in several ways:

- Cart Fill

- ADM (Automated Dispensing Machines)

- Reorders (if not in cart fill or the ADM)

Cart Fill   In a cart fill system, each patient has a cassette (drawer that is labeled for them and contains a set supply of that day's medications). In addition, there is a second cassette for the patient in the pharmacy that is for *tomorrow's* doses. These cassettes are usually exchanged every 24 hours (sometimes twice a day, sometimes every other day). *Filling and exchanging cassettes is a primary technician duty.*

Unlike retail prescriptions, hospital patients' prescriptions change often since patients are much more acutely ill and their conditions change so often from procedures and surgeries in the hospitals. As orders change throughout the day, medications are added and removed from the patient's cassette.

It is important to know how many doses to dispense. Orders are written to be **scheduled** (given at set times) or **PRN** (given as needed per the parameters of the order). For instance a medication ordered twice a day (BID) is to be given regularly, twice a day. A PRN order, however, is only given if the conditions exist as ordered and a PRN order should always include a condition (such as pain, insomnia, constipation, etc.). For instance, a medication ordered as "BIDPRN PAIN" can be given *up to* twice a day and only if the patient has pain. No more than two doses can be given a day, and if the patient still has pain, a new order must be received from the physician. Assuming a 24-hour supply of medication is to be dispensed, you would dispense two doses for both of these orders (BID and BIDPRN pain).

ADM (Automated Dispensing Machines)   ADMs (Pyxis, Omnicell, etc.) are machines that have computers that restrict access via passwords to authorized users. The machines contain drawers and compartments filled with *medications that are not patient specific.* These medications include prescription drugs, over-the-counter drugs, and controlled substances. Each drug has a minimum and maximum level and requires the user (usually the nurse) to access the machine and enter removals for each patient. As removals are entered, the ADM keeps track of the doses removed and when the amount left in the ADM reaches the minimum level, a report is generated to refill the ADM. *Refilling of ADMs is another primary technician function.*

Sometimes the ADM allows the user to remove any drug for any patient; other times the ADM only allows the user to remove drugs that are specifically ordered for that patient.

Reorders   Reorders are like new orders in that the pharmacy needs to dispense the medication separately from the ADM or the cart fill. This can be in the case of a **multidose item** (an item that contains more than one dose) such as a bottle of eye drops or a tube of a cream or ointment and for which the initial supply has been lost or used up. Reorders can also be used for **single-dose medications** (a container that has only one individual dose or which can only be used one time). Multidose items often have a preservative that helps retard bacterial growth. Single-dose medications typically contain no preservative and are labeled for one-time use only. Regardless of the type of medication, a new supply is sent to the nursing unit for the patient.

Bar-coding   Increasingly, hospital pharmacies are utilizing bar codes on medications to insure patient safety. Bar codes can either be ones that drug manufacturers put directly on the individual products or ones that the pharmacy generates on the product or the patient label. In the bar-coding system, when the nurse goes to give a patient a dose, the drug, nurse name badge, and the patient bar code are all scanned to make sure the correct drug is given.

This bar-code system is related to the patient safety initiative called the **5 Rs**: the right drug, the right dose, to the right patient, in the right amount at the right time. **The 5 Rs is the ultimate goal of all hospital pharmacies and of the unit dose system.**

In addition, some pharmacies use bar-coding to receive drugs coming into the pharmacy and to refill the ADM. If bar-coding is not used for ADM refilling, mistakes can be made by the technician. **It should be noted that it is always important for technicians to double-check themselves in all the work they do.**

Labeling and Storage   Pharmacy staff, including technicians, are responsible for the proper storage and labeling of medications. Storage includes refrigerated drugs, drugs that need light protection, drugs that need to be locked up (controlled substances), and drugs that are within the manufacturer's expiration date. There are a number of labels attached to drugs, not only for storage conditions but also for such things as drugs requiring filtration, drugs that should not be crushed or chewed, drugs with special administration instructions, and the like. Pharmacy technicians need to be familiar with all drugs that require special handling and storage.

Drug Packaging   Unit dose oral solid-drug packaging can be done via machine or via hand systems called bubble packs. Oral liquids are packaged in bottles, unit dose cups, or oral syringes (for children). In all cases, the package must be labeled with <u>at least</u>:

- Drug generic name

- Drug trade name (may be most common trade name)

- Dosage form (tablet, capsule, etc.)

- Strength or concentration (for liquids)

- Volume (liquids only)

- Lot number

- Expiration date (usually a maximum of one year if packaged)

- In addition, there may be other information required such as: "chemotherapy" or "extended release" depending on the medication being repackaged.

PRACTICE EXERCISE 1 ──────────────────────────────────────

1. You are given some handwritten orders and a manual (handwritten) patient profile. Transcribe the physician orders to the patient profile, including the amount you would dispense for a 24-hour supply (level).

2. Describe what required element is missing from the following sample drug package label.

```
┌─────────────────────────────────────┐
│                                      │
│            Acetaminophen             │
│                                      │
│             (Tylenol)                │
│                                      │
│              325mg                   │
│                                      │
│   Lot # 12345      Exp Date 9-09     │
│                                      │
└─────────────────────────────────────┘
```

_____

_____

_____

3. Which of the following is NOT one of the "5 Rs"?

   a. Right dose

   b. Right time

   c. Right patient

   d. Right price

4. Which is NOT a primary duty of pharmacy technicians in hospitals?

   a. Refilling of ADMs

   b. Cart filling

   c. Reviewing new medication orders for correctness

5. Name two ways that pharmacies typically fill standing orders for medications.

   a. _____

   b. _____

6. What are the two main types of orders that hospital pharmacies dispense?

   a. _____

   b. _____

7. Name two methods that hospitals use to transcribe medication orders.

   a. _____

   b. _____

INJECTABLE MEDICATIONS

Injectable medications can be given to patients in multiple ways:

IM	intramuscular—such as a shot in the arm
SC	subcutaneous—under the skin
IT	intrathecal—delivered into the spinal fluid
Epidural	delivered into the space between disks of the spine

IV   intravenous—delivered into the vein

IA   intra-arterial—delivered into an artery

Medications given IM or SC are most commonly dispensed as vials, dispensed from the unit dose area and drawn up by nurses. Medications given IV, IT, Epidural are most commonly made in a pharmacy IV compounding room. IV medications can be given as:

LVP Large Volume Parenteral, volume usually >250mls and usually given continuously into IV tubing

SVP Small Volume Parenterals, also called IV piggybacks, volume usually <250mls and given intermittently into the IV tubing of another IV

The compounding of all of these medications is another of the primary functions of hospital-based pharmacy technicians. These medications are prepared according to the physician order and compounding guidelines related to physical compatibility (if things can be mixed together) and stability (how long something lasts once it is mixed).

Compounding is done aseptically (in such a way to eliminate bacteria) in the pharmacy. Only sterile items from drug manufacturers are used to compound these items. Technicians are tasked with doing their own calculations on how much of a drug is needed to compound the needed items. Drug concentrations (how much of a drug is in how many milliliters [mls] of the drug in solution) can either be on the drug vial (drugs that come in solutions) or from reconstituting a powder into solution (also listed on the drug vial). It is important for technicians to always use calculators and to double-check themselves before compounding an item.

Premixes There are a number of commercially available premixed products that do not require pharmacy admixture. These premixed IV solutions contain one additive to a base IV solution and can be LVPs or SVPs. Because of stability issues, there are also a number of IV systems for SVPs in which the drug and diluent can be attached or mixed with each other without actual pharmacy admixture.

IV Aseptic Technique

Aseptic technique is a method of compounding that tries to minimize or eliminate the possibility of bacteria being introduced into products being compounded and administered into IV lines of patients (where great harm can be done to already sick patients). There are national guidelines on how best to do this (called USP 797). In simplest terms, the way to minimize bacteria is to minimize the risk of touch contamination (bacteria introduced via our hands) or airborne contamination (bacteria that attaches to airborne particles and contaminates IVs being compounded).

USP guidelines call for the following:

- A positive pressure clean room, where the air is constantly recirculated through HEPA filters (filters that screen out very small particles)

- Strict gowning procedures for covering clothes, hair, and shoes so as to minimize particles and dirt from the outside

- Strict guidelines for removing jewelry, flaky make-up, and the length of fingernails, all of which carry bacteria

- Thorough hand-washing, the wearing of gloves, and the constant cleaning of gloves

- Compounding only in IV hoods, where the air is further put through HEPA filters

- The regular cleaning with germicides of the room and all the items in it, including the floors, walls, and ceiling and all the drugs and IV solutions

- The regular testing of samples made in the compounding room to assure that they are sterile

If a clean room is not available, USP guidelines allow IVs to be made in an IV room where the air is not filtered, but the IVs must be made in a closed glove box-type hood.

Compounding of IV products is based on the physician order that has been reviewed by the pharmacist for appropriateness, compatibility, and other issues. After this process, a label is produced upon which the IV is to be compounded.

A properly composed label must have the following components:

- Patient name

- Patient location (bed number)

- Drug(s) to be added (additives)

- Base solution (the primary IV solution used to dilute the drugs)

- A rate or administration time (how quickly the solution is to be given)

- An expiration date (and often the compounded date and time)

- The initials of the person who made it and who checked it

The technician then assembles the items needed to compound, including syringes, needles, alcohol pads (to swab all the items on which bacteria might be present), and the drugs and IV solution. The IV is then made and checked by a pharmacist. Because of time constraints, the IV is often checked long after it is made, so the technician leaves all the items needed to be checked:

- Any drug vials used, marked as to concentration

- Any syringes used and pulled back to the volume used for each drug vial

- The IV solution used

- The IV label

Chemotherapy   Chemotherapy (anti-neo-plastic) medications are drugs used to treat cancer. These same drugs that can treat cancer are very toxic and can even cause harm to healthy individuals. So that workers compounding chemotherapy are protected, chemotherapy IV medications must be compounded in a hood designated for that purpose and whose air is vented outside of the room. In addition, special items are used to prevent spills and special protective gloves and gowns are worn to further protect the person compounding chemotherapy. All of these items are disposed of in specially marked containers to prevent any other accidental exposure.

OTHER TECHNICIAN FUNCTIONS

Pharmacy technicians perform a number of other functions in the pharmacy such as:

- Drug ordering and receiving from outside vendors

- Stocking of supplies and drugs on shelves

- Checking for outdated drugs throughout the hospital

- Packaging drugs

- Compounding drugs, not commercially available

- Answering telephones and providing other services such as delivering medications

- Billing patients

Pharmacy technicians have proved a valuable asset in the hospital pharmacy setting and indeed it is hard to imagine hospitals without them. Medication safety continues to evolve and become ever more important to medical practice. So too do the ever-growing number and complexity of medications put ever-increasing demands on pharmacies to provide services and information about medications. As the profession of pharmacy continues to grow and expand in the hospital setting, so too does the role of pharmacy technicians. For instance, in some states, technicians are allowed to check the work of other technicians (under carefully limited circumstances appropriate to pharmacy technicians' abilities and education). The future of pharmacy technicians is one of respect and growing possibilities.

PRACTICE EXERCISE 2 ─────────────────────────────

1. You are asked to make an IV piggyback of Gentamicin 60mg in Dextrose 5% 50ml. You are given a vial of Gentamicin 40mg/mls, 2mls. How many mls do you need to make 60mg?

_____

_____

_____

2. For the following drugs, how much is needed to give the shown amount?

   Sodium Acetate 4mEq/ml   28mEq = _____mls

   Cefazolin 10mg/ml   500mgs = _____mls

   Dopamine 80mg/ml   400mg = _____ mls

3. What is missing from this improperly composed IV label?

John Smith Bed	456-A
Potassium Chloride	
In	
Dextrose 5% in 0.45% Sodium Chloride	1000 ml
Administer over 30 minutes	
Expiration: 9-9-08	
Compounded: 9-8-08	
Made by: XX	Checked by: YY

_____

_____

_____

4. USP guidelines for IV compounding require which of the following?

   a. Compounding of IVs in a hood

   b. The regular cleaning of all items in the clean room

   c. Gowns, shoe covers, gloves, and hair covers

   d. A sterile field

5. What do the following abbreviations stand for?

   IM _____

   IV _____

   PR _____

6. What are the four required items that technicians must leave for a pharmacist to check their work in the IV room?

   a. _____

   b. _____

   c. _____

   d. _____

7. If you have a 500ml IV bag of sodium chloride 0.9%, is that an SVP or an LVP?

_____

MAR INSTRUCTIONS ——————————————————————

Using the provided medication administration record, transfer the physician's order information to the MAR. Using the blank physician's order sheet, the student will complete his/her own order and give it to a classmate in order to fill out a MAR. You will also be required to keep an inventory of what medications were dispensed to the nursing stations. When deciding what medications to give, refer to the Unit Dose Formulary provided. Complete a Unit Dose Tracking sheet for each patient. List the remaining amount of repacked medications available once the order has been filled. If there is not enough medication for dispensing, calculate how many units are needed to fill the order.

   Example, if the order is written as

   Order: Amoxil 500mg qd

   Stock on hand: Amoxil 250mg

The patient is to receive two tablets of Amoxil 250mg per dose. See sample tracking sheet for more help.

Unit Dose Formulary

Name	Strength	Lot #	Exp. Date	Amount on hand
Acetaminophen	0.5gm	ACE05	06/2077	35
Acetaminophen	0.375gm	ACE375	06/2077	14
Acetaminophen	0.65gm	SUPP	06/2077	10
Actos	0.015gm	ACT15	09/2025	6
Actos	0.03gm	ACT33	09/2020	5
Amoxil	0.25gm	AMO5	09/2020	3
Aspirin	0.081gm	ASA44	12/2020	5
Atorvastatin Ca	0.10gm	ATO10	12/2020	2
Atorvastatin Ca	0.20gm	ATO20	12/2020	6
Bisulfate	0.075gm	CLOB75	07/2019	5
Cephalexin	0.33gm	CEP33	09/2066	5
Cephalexin	0.50gm	CEP50	09/2066	2
Ciprofloxacin	0.75gm	CIP75	04/2058	8
Ciprofloxacin	0.5gm	CIP50	06/2080	10
Clopidogrel	0.075g	CLO075	06/2044	10
Digitek	125mcg	DIG125	12/2022	6
Diphenhydramine	0.025gm	DIP55	01/2026	10
Docusate Sodium	0.25gm	DOC5	01/2105	8
Dulcolax	Supp	DUL	04/2044	6
Hydrocodone Bitartrate and Acetaminophen	5/500	HYAC	06/2011	10
Hydrocodone Bitartrate and Acetaminophen	7.5/750	HYES	06/2011	15
Ibuprofen	0.6gm	IBU6	02/2088	9
Ibuprofen	0.08gm	IBU8	02/2088	12
Indinavir Sulfate	0.33gm	IND33	03/2088	13
Indinavir Sulfate	0.04gm	IND04	03/2055	11
Metformin	0.85gm	MET85	03/2012	12
Metformin	1000mg	MET00	03/2012	10
MOM	———	MOM	03/2112	60ml

Name	Strength	Lot #	Exp. Date	Amount on hand
Maalox	15ml	MAA15	08/2022	15ml
Maalox	30ml	MAA30	08/2022	30ml
Penicillin V	0.25gm	PEN25	08/2022	6
Potassium	0.250gm	PEN25	03/2045	8
Principen	0.5gm	PRIN11	10/2020	3
Principen	0.2gm	PRIN22	05/2036	2
Prochlorperazine	0.01gm	PRO10	05/2025	4
Prochlorperazine	0.05gm	PRO5	05/2025	5
Proventil HFA	———	PVTL	04/2033	4
Ritonavir	0.1gm	RET100	05/2025	12
Rosiglitazone	0.02gm	ROS2	04/2030	10
Rosiglitazone	0.08gm	ROS8	04/2055	10
Saquinavir Mesylate	0.5gm	SAQ500	08/2022	10
Tears Natural	———	TND	02/2011	3 bottles
Tenormin	0.010gm	TEN10	05/2075	12
Tiazac	0.015gm	TIA15	02/2012	6
Trandolapril	1mg	TRA1	11/2011	8
Trandolapril	2mg	TRA2	12/2012	3
Vasotec	0.0025gm	VAS25	06/2022	5
Vasotec	0.01gm	VAS10	06/2022	5

PHYSICIAN'S ORDERS

PLEASE USE BALLPOINT PEN AND PRESS HARD

DRUG SENSITIVITY

| DATE 9-8-08 | TIME 14:25 | AUTHORIZATION IS GIVEN TO DISPENSE GENERIC EQUIVALENT UNLESS CHECKED HERE | ▸ ☐ |

R.N.

Acetaminophen 325mg po q4h prn pain
Maalox 30ml po Bid prn indigestion
Lipitor 10mg po qd
Digoxin 0.125mg po qd
Cipro 500mg po q12h
Diltiazem 30mg po q6h
Morphine 2mg IV q3h prn pain
Acetaminophen 650mg suppos. rectally q6h prn
temp > 38.5

John Smith   Bed 456-A
Date of Birth: 3-4-72
Acct #0055555   MR#0000078
Attending MD: Dr Mary Cooper

| DATE | TIME | AUTHORIZATION IS GIVEN TO DISPENSE GENERIC EQUIVALENT UNLESS CHECKED HERE | ▸ ☐ |

R.N.

John Smith   Bed 456-A
Date of Birth: 3-4-72
Acct #0055555   MR#0000078
Attending MD: Dr Mary Cooper

| DATE | TIME | AUTHORIZATION IS GIVEN TO DISPENSE GENERIC EQUIVALENT UNLESS CHECKED HERE | ▸ ☐ |

R.N.

John Smith   Bed 456-A
Date of Birth: 3-4-72
Acct #0055555   MR#0000078
Attending MD: Dr Mary Cooper

FORM F-1119A (REV. 6/05)

PHYSICIAN'S ORDERS

Table 19-1

Allergies: Mr #   Date of Birth:

Diagnosis: Attending MD: Name: John Smith   Rm #

HOSPITAL MAR

DATE:

START / STOP	MEDICATION AND STRENGTH	FORM	DOSING SCHEDULE	# DISP	# ON HAND	TECH R.Ph										

PHYSICIAN'S ORDERS

PLEASE USE BALLPOINT PEN AND PRESS HARD

DRUG SENSITIVITY

DATE 8-15-08	TIME 12:30	AUTHORIZATION IS GIVEN TO DISPENSE GENERIC EQUIVALENT UNLESS CHECKED HERE	➡ ☐	
				R.N.

Admit patient to 5th Floor

Docusate sodium 100mg BID

Milk of Magnesia 30ml qd prn constipation

Bisacodyl Suppos. pr prn constipation

Vicodin ÷ po q6h prn mild pain

Vicodin ++ po q6h prn severe pain

Start IV D5 1/2 + 20 Kcl @ 125ml /hr

Ampicillin 1gm IVPB q6h

Albuterol inhaler ÷ puff q4h prn respiratory distress

James Smith Bed 555-5
DOB: 6-6-70
Dr. Wayne Doe
MR#4445550 Acct #00088897

DATE	TIME	AUTHORIZATION IS GIVEN TO DISPENSE GENERIC EQUIVALENT UNLESS CHECKED HERE	➡ ☐	
				R.N.

Tears Naturale ÷ gtt OU prn dry eyes

diagnosis: Pneumonia

Height 6'1", weight 190 lbs.

Allergies — none

Diet: regular

James Smith Bed 555-5
DOB: 6-6-70
Dr. Wayne Doe
MR#4445550 Acct #00088897

DATE	TIME	AUTHORIZATION IS GIVEN TO DISPENSE GENERIC EQUIVALENT UNLESS CHECKED HERE	➡ ☐	
				R.N.

James Smith Bed 555-5
DOB: 6-6-70
Dr. Wayne Doe
MR#4445550 Acct #00088897

PHYSICIAN'S ORDERS

PHARMACY 1

Table 19-2

Allergies: Mr #   Date of Birth:

Diagnosis: Attending MD: Name: James Smith   Rm #

HOSPITAL MAR

START / STOP	MEDICATION AND STRENGTH	FORM	DOSING SCHEDULE	# DISP	# ON HAND	TECH R.Ph	DATE:										

Please use BLACK ink only

ADVENTURE HOSPITAL

Physician Order Sheet

Drug Allergies: NKDA   DX: Diabetic / HBP

Date: 8/8	Generic equivalent allowed if checked here ☑

pt admitted @ 1325 to Rm 1111A
history of diabetes & kidney damage
D5W 1 liter 50ml/hrs
Glucophage 500mg ī qam
Actos 15mg ī qd
Mavik 4mg ī qhs
Enalapril 0mg ī qam

DR. Mundian

Jack Flarious   Bed 1111A
Date of Birth: 01/11/xx   Age: 45
MR# 965843
Attending Physician: Dr. Kim Mundian

Date: 8/9	Generic equivalent allowed if checked here ☑

pt. feeling nausea/vomit.
compazine rect. supp 25mg
q 4hrs prn
Tylenol 0.5gm q 4hrs T>101°
Continue all meds
@ 1430
DR Mundian

Jack Flarious   Bed 1111A
Date of Birth: 01/11/xx   Age: 45
MR# 965843
Attending Physician: Dr. Kim Mundian

Date: 8/10	Generic equivalent allowed if checked here ☐

Sugar level increased
Δ Glucophage to 0.1gm qam
D/C actos
Δ to Avandia 4mg ī qd
pt. doing well
re-evaluated @ 1500 hrs

Pt. can be discharged

DR. Mundian

Jack Flarious   Bed 1111A
Date of Birth: 01/11/xx   Age: 45
MR# 965843
Attending Physician: Dr. Kim Mundian

Form # 060975

Rev 10/08

Table 19-3

Allergies:

Diagnosis:

Date of Birth:

Mr #

Name: Jack Flarious

Attending MD:

Rm #

HOSPITAL MAR

START / STOP	MEDICATION AND STRENGTH	FORM	DOSING SCHEDULE	# DISP	# ON HAND	TECH R.Ph	DATE:										

Please use BLACK ink only

ADVENTURE HOSPITAL
Physician Order Sheet

Drug Allergies: TCN	DX: Resp. infec. / HIV +

Date: 12/12   Generic equivalent allowed if checked here ☑

Admitted to 777A @ 0600
pt. has severe resp. problems/HIV+
PCN 500mg ī q 4 hrs
Benadryl 50mg ī q 12 hrs
Crixivan 0.4gm īī q 8 hrs w/
Norvir 0.1gm īī bid (80) īī bid
D5WNS in 2.4L @ 100mL/24hrs
× 3d
                    DR. Diver

Attending Physician: Dr. Skye Diver   MR# 777666   Date of Birth: 07/07/xx   Age: 56   Bed 777A   Abra Cadabra

Date: 12/13   Generic equivalent allowed if checked here ☑

pt doing well w/ resp infection
present w/ HIV complications (0800)
D/C Benadryl
Δ PCN to Keflex 500mg ī q 4 hrs
Continue w/ meds, add
Invirase 0.5gm īī bid
Morphine 2mg IV q 3 hrs prn pain
VS q 2 hrs ATC
                    DR Diver

Attending Physician: Dr. Skye Diver   MR# 777666   Date of Birth: 07/07/xx   Age: 56   Bed 777A   Abra Cadabra

Date: 12/14   Generic equivalent allowed if checked here ☑

pt. stable HIV complications
still present.
        Continue all meds
D5WNS in 2.4L @ 100ml/hr
continous
Re-evaluate   DR. Diver
@ 1000 DD

Attending Physician: Dr. Skye Diver   MR# 777666   Date of Birth: 07/07/xx   Age: 56   Bed 777A   Abra Cadabra

Physician Order Sheet

Form # 060975

Rev 10/08

Table 19-4

Allergies:

Diagnosis:

Mr #

Attending MD:

Date of Birth:

Name: Abra Cadabra

Rm #

HOSPITAL MAR

START / STOP	MEDICATION AND STRENGTH	FORM	DOSING SCHEDULE	# DISP	# ON HAND	TECH R.Ph	DATE:										

Please use BLACK ink only

ADVENTURE HOSPITAL	
Physician Order Sheet	

Drug Allergies: PCN	DX: Angina Pectoris	

Date: 4/30 — Generic equivalent allowed if checked here ☑

admitted @ 1500 hrs. Pt complain
of chest pain, history of heart prob.
ASA 81mg ī qd
Plavix 75mg ī qd
Cipro 500mg ī q 4hrs
VS q 4 hrs
Motrin 600mg ī q 12hrs prn pain
D5W ½ NS in 1 liter @ 100 ml/hr
continous   DR. Dhillon

*Pretty Boy   Bed 666A
Date of Birth: 02/17/xx   Age: 30
MR# 124578
Attending Physician:Dr. Raji Dhillon*

Date: — Generic equivalent allowed if checked here ☑

Re evaluated @ 1700 hrs
pt stable
D/C Cipro 500mg
Continue all meds, add
Compazine supp. 25mg prn n/v
atenolol 25mg ī qhs
                DR Dhillon

*Pretty Boy   Bed 666A
Date of Birth: 02/17/xx   Age: 30
MR# 124578
Attending Physician:Dr. Raji Dhillon*

Date: 5/2 — Generic equivalent allowed if checked here ☑

pt in good condition
D/C @ 1900 hrs
atenolol 25mg ī qhs X30
Plavix 75mg ī qd X30
ASA 81mg ī qd X30
                DR. Dhillon

*Pretty Boy   Bed 666A
Date of Birth: 02/17/xx   Age: 30
MR# 124578
Attending Physician:Dr. Raji Dhillon*

Physician Order Sheet

Form # 060975

Rev 10/08

Table 19-5

Allergies:

Diagnosis:

Mr #

Attending MD:

Date of Birth:

Name: Pretty Boy

Rm #

HOSPITAL MAR

DATE:

START / STOP	MEDICATION AND STRENGTH	FORM	DOSING SCHEDULE	# DISP	# ON HAND	TECH R.Ph												

PHYSICIAN'S ORDERS

PLEASE USE BALLPOINT PEN AND PRESS HARD

DRUG SENSITIVITY

DATE	TIME	AUTHORIZATION IS GIVEN TO DISPENSE GENERIC EQUIVALENT UNLESS CHECKED HERE		
				R.N.

DATE	TIME	AUTHORIZATION IS GIVEN TO DISPENSE GENERIC EQUIVALENT UNLESS CHECKED HERE		
				R.N.

DATE	TIME	AUTHORIZATION IS GIVEN TO DISPENSE GENERIC EQUIVALENT UNLESS CHECKED HERE		
				R.N.

PHYSICIAN'S ORDERS

PHARMACY 1

Table 19-6

Allergies: Mr #   Date of Birth:

Diagnosis: Attending MD: Name: Rm #

HOSPITAL MAR

START / STOP	MEDICATION AND STRENGTH	FORM	DOSING SCHEDULE	# DISP	# ON HAND	TECH R.Ph	DATE:										

TPN INSTRUCTIONS

Using the TPN orders provided (page 169) calculate the following:

1. Total mEq/day

2. Total mEq/dose

3. Total ml/bag needed

Additional TPN orders can be found in the Appendix.

Please use BLACK ink only

ADVENTURE HOSPITAL	
Physician Order Sheet	

Drug Allergies: PCN

Date: 3-3 | Generic equivalent allowed if checked here ☐

Wt @ 135 lbs   DX: IBS, Malnutrition

Calcium   12 mEq ⎫
KCL   70 mEq   ⎬ q 24 hrs
Chloride   10 mEq ⎭

3.6 NS
0.9 over
24 hrs
(PL)

Chana

TPN 1

Date: 3-4 | Generic equivalent allowed if checked here ☐

Wt 225 lb   NS 0.9% 2.4 L
(CL) over 24 hrs

MVI   10 mL   Dx: Abscess
KCL   80 mEq   Allergies: Amoxil
Insulin   10 u
Zinc   2.5 mg

SBomgal

TPN 2

Date: 3-5 | Generic equivalent allowed if checked here ☐

Wt 333 lb   DX: Diverticulous
Copper 3mg   Allergy: Colace
Magnesium   16 mEq
Calcium 12 mEq
Sodium 20 mEq

NS 0.225% 6L   over 24 hrs
over 24 hrs
(PC)

SBomgal

TPN 3

Form # 060975

Rev 10/08

Please use BLACK ink only

ADVENTURE HOSPITAL

Physician Order Sheet

Drug Allergies:	TCN, Sulfa

Date: Generic equivalent allowed if checked here ☐

Wt 701 lbs   DX: Pancreatitis

Δ amino acid to 3 Gm/kg

Δ Dextrose to 8 Gm/kg

Calcium 80 mEq

Zinc 5mg   over 24 hrs

3L DNS over

24 hrs PL   SBangal

TPN 4

Date: Generic equivalent allowed if checked here ☐

Wt 275 lb   4.8 L NS½ over 24hrs

Δ Lipids to 2 Gm/kg (PL)

Calcium 70 mEq

Magnesium 15 mEq

Copper 10 mg

R Mundian

NKDA   DX: Fistula

TPN 5

Date: Generic equivalent allowed if checked here ☐

Wt 525 lb   NS 150 mL/hr over (CL)

~~Selenide~~ Ⓓ   24 hrs

Magnesium 3 mEq   DX:

~~Cromium~~ Ⓓ   Short

Chromium 10 mg   Bowel

mVI 15 mls   NKDA

KCL 90 mEq

Dhillon, R.

TPN 6

Form # 060975

Rev 10/08

Please use BLACK ink only

ADVENTURE HOSPITAL	
Physician Order Sheet	

Drug Allergies:	Iodine, Cipro	

Date:	Generic equivalent allowed if checked here ☐	TPN 7
Zinc 5mg Wt: 380 lbs Copper 1mg KCL 80 mEq } qd Calcium 12mEq LVP NS ½ 5.4 L over 24hrs. Dx: Ileus (PL) Radia Dx: Inflammatory Bowel disease		

Date:	Generic equivalent allowed if checked here ☐	TPN 8
Calcium 14mEq Wt: 100 lbs Insulin 30 u Zinc 5mg } over 24hrs Copper 12mg MVI 4mls NS 0.9% 1.8 L over 24hrs (PL) Dx: Malabsorption Dhillon		

Date:	Generic equivalent allowed if checked here ☐	TPN 9
Wt 175lb Dx: maldigestion Chromium 15mg KCL 20 mEq Calcium 80mEq Zinc 4mg NS ½ 1.56 L over 24 hrs (CL) Chana		

Form # 060975

Rev 10/08

Please use BLACK ink only

ADVENTURE HOSPITAL
Physician Order Sheet

Drug Allergies:	Keflex, Calcium	

Date:	Generic equivalent allowed if checked here ☐	TPN 10
	Wt: 200 lbs Magnesium 5mEq KCL 80mEq } qd Sodium 40mEq Calcium 12mEq NS 0.9% 150mls for 24hrs (PL) DX: Fistula/abscess De Bangaf	

Date:	Generic equivalent allowed if checked here ☐	TPN 11
	Wt: 150lb NS ¼ @ 135mL/hr KCL 40mEq over 5hrs (PL) Calcium 24mEq ~~D5NS 100mls over 24hrs~~ D/C Bangaf DX: Bowel Obstruction NKDA	

Date:	Generic equivalent allowed if checked here ☐	TPN 12
	Wt: 125lb DX: Short Bowel NS 0.9% 35mL/hr for 6hrs (CL) ~~c~~ Calcium 12mEq Chromium 20mg Sodium 80mEq KCL 40mEq NS 125mL/hr over 8hrs NKDA Diver, S.	

Form # 060975

Rev 10/08

ADVENTURE HOSPITAL
TPN PHARMACY ORDER

Patient Name _____

Allergies _____

MR # _____

Calculate the amount of grams needed per day for the standard formula; calculate the ml to be given per liter for the additives. Complete one TPN pharmacy order for each day per patient

Indication for TPN: _____ Wt: _____

Route: ☐ Central Line (CL)   ☐ Peripheral Line (PL)

Date: _____

Flow Rate _____ ml/hr, Total ml/day _____, Total L/day _____

Standard Formula:	Recommended Dosage	Per Day
Amino Acids	4GM/kg	_____ GM
Dextrose	1.5GM/kg	_____ GM
Lipids	1GM/kg	_____ GM

Additives (available stock):		Per Dose	Per Dose
KCl	(40mEq/50ml)	_____ mEq	_____ ml
NaAcetate	(40mEq/ml)	_____ mEq	_____ ml
CaGluconate	(45mEq/ml)	_____ mEq	_____ ml
MgSO$_4$	(5mEq/2.5ml)	_____ mEq	_____ ml
Multivit Conc.	———	_____ ml	_____ ml
Zn	(1mg/ml)	_____ mg	_____ ml
Cu	(0.4mg/ml)	_____ mg	_____ ml
Mn	(4mg/3ml)	_____ mg	_____ ml
Cr	(4mcg/ml)	_____ mg	_____ ml
Insulin		_____ U	_____ ml

STANDARD PHARMACY ORDERS:
Always compound TPN / IV using aseptic technique

Pharmacy Technician Name: _____

Pharmacy Technician Signature: _____

Date: _____

ADVENTURE HOSPITAL
TPN PHARMACY ORDER

Patient Name _____

Allergies _____

MR # _____

Calculate the amount of grams needed per day for the standard formula; calculate the ml to be given per liter for the additives. Complete one TPN pharmacy order for each day per patient

Indication for TPN: _____ Wt: _____

Route: ☐ Central Line (CL)   ☐ Peripheral Line (PL)

Date: _____

Flow Rate _____ ml/hr, Total ml/day _____, Total L/day _____

Standard Formula:	Recommended Dosage	Per Day
Amino Acids	4GM/kg	_____ GM
Dextrose	1.5GM/kg	_____ GM
Lipids	1GM/kg	_____ GM

Additives (available stock):		Per Dose	Per Dose
KCl	(40mEq/50ml)	_____ mEq	_____ ml
NaAcetate	(40mEq/ml)	_____ mEq	_____ ml
CaGluconate	(45mEq/ml)	_____ mEq	_____ ml
MgSO$_4$	(5mEq/2.5ml)	_____ mEq	_____ ml
Multivit Conc.	———	_____ ml	_____ ml
Zn	(1mg/ml)	_____ mg	_____ ml
Cu	(0.4mg/ml)	_____ mg	_____ ml
Mn	(4mg/3ml)	_____ mg	_____ ml
Cr	(4mcg/ml)	_____ mg	_____ ml
Insulin		_____ U	_____ ml

STANDARD PHARMACY ORDERS:
Always compound TPN / IV using aseptic technique

Pharmacy Technician Name: _____

Pharmacy Technician Signature: _____

Date: _____

ADVENTURE HOSPITAL
TPN PHARMACY ORDER

Patient Name _____

Allergies _____

MR # _____

Calculate the amount of grams needed per day for the standard formula; calculate the ml to be given per liter for the additives. Complete one TPN pharmacy order for each day per patient

Indication for TPN: _____ Wt: _____

Route: ☐ Central Line (CL)   ☐ Peripheral Line (PL)

Date: _____

Flow Rate _____ ml/hr, Total ml/day _____, Total L/day _____

Standard Formula:	Recommended Dosage	Per Day
Amino Acids	4GM/kg	_____ GM
Dextrose	1.5GM/kg	_____ GM
Lipids	1GM/kg	_____ GM

Additives (available stock):		Per Dose	Per Dose
KCl	(40mEq/50ml)	_____ mEq	_____ ml
NaAcetate	(40mEq/ml)	_____ mEq	_____ ml
CaGluconate	(45mEq/ml)	_____ mEq	_____ ml
$MgSO_4$	(5mEq/2.5ml)	_____ mEq	_____ ml
Multivit Conc.	———	_____ ml	_____ ml
Zn	(1mg/ml)	_____ mg	_____ ml
Cu	(0.4mg/ml)	_____ mg	_____ ml
Mn	(4mg/3ml)	_____ mg	_____ ml
Cr	(4mcg/ml)	_____ mg	_____ ml
Insulin		_____ U	_____ ml

STANDARD PHARMACY ORDERS:
Always compound TPN / IV using aseptic technique

Pharmacy Technician Name: _____

Pharmacy Technician Signature: _____

Date: _____

ADVENTURE HOSPITAL
TPN PHARMACY ORDER

Patient Name _____

Allergies _____

MR # _____

Calculate the amount of grams needed per day for the standard formula; calculate the ml to be given per liter for the additives. Complete one TPN pharmacy order for each day per patient

Indication for TPN: _____ Wt: _____

Route: ☐ Central Line (CL) ☐ Peripheral Line (PL)

Date: _____

Flow Rate _____ ml/hr, Total ml/day _____, Total L/day _____

Standard Formula:	Recommended Dosage	Per Day
Amino Acids	4GM/kg	_____ GM
Dextrose	1.5GM/kg	_____ GM
Lipids	1GM/kg	_____ GM

Additives (available stock):		Per Dose	Per Dose
KCl	(40mEq/50ml)	_____ mEq	_____ ml
NaAcetate	(40mEq/ml)	_____ mEq	_____ ml
CaGluconate	(45mEq/ml)	_____ mEq	_____ ml
$MgSO_4$	(5mEq/2.5ml)	_____ mEq	_____ ml
Multivit Conc.	———	_____ ml	_____ ml
Zn	(1mg/ml)	_____ mg	_____ ml
Cu	(0.4mg/ml)	_____ mg	_____ ml
Mn	(4mg/3ml)	_____ mg	_____ ml
Cr	(4mcg/ml)	_____ mg	_____ ml
Insulin		_____ U	_____ ml

STANDARD PHARMACY ORDERS:
Always compound TPN / IV using aseptic technique

Pharmacy Technician Name: _____

Pharmacy Technician Signature: _____

Date: _____

ADVENTURE HOSPITAL
TPN PHARMACY ORDER

Patient Name   _____

Allergies _____

MR #   _____

Calculate the amount of grams needed per day for the standard formula; calculate the ml to be given per liter for the additives. Complete one TPN pharmacy order for each day per patient

Indication for TPN: _____ **Wt:** _____

Route: ☐ **Central Line (CL)**   ☐ **Peripheral Line (PL)**

Date: _____

Flow Rate _____ ml/hr, Total ml/day _____, Total L/day _____

Standard Formula:	Recommended Dosage	Per Day
Amino Acids	4GM/kg	_____ GM
Dextrose	1.5GM/kg	_____ GM
Lipids	1GM/kg	_____ GM

Additives (available stock):		Per Dose	Per Dose
KCl	(40mEq/50ml)	_____ mEq	_____ ml
NaAcetate	(40mEq/ml)	_____ mEq	_____ ml
CaGluconate	(45mEq/ml)	_____ mEq	_____ ml
MgSO$_4$	(5mEq/2.5ml)	_____ mEq	_____ ml
Multivit Conc.	_____	_____ ml	_____ ml
Zn	(1mg/ml)	_____ mg	_____ ml
Cu	(0.4mg/ml)	_____ mg	_____ ml
Mn	(4mg/3ml)	_____ mg	_____ ml
Cr	(4mcg/ml)	_____ mg	_____ ml
Insulin		_____ U	_____ ml

STANDARD PHARMACY ORDERS:
Always compound TPN / IV using aseptic technique

Pharmacy Technician Name: _____

Pharmacy Technician Signature: _____

Date: _____

ADVENTURE HOSPITAL
TPN PHARMACY ORDER

Patient Name _____

Allergies _____

MR # _____

Calculate the amount of grams needed per day for the standard formula; calculate the ml to be given per liter for the additives. Complete one TPN pharmacy order for each day per patient

Indication for TPN: _____ Wt: _____

Route: ☐ Central Line (CL)   ☐ Peripheral Line (PL)

Date: _____

Flow Rate _____ ml/hr, Total ml/day _____, Total L/day _____

Standard Formula:	Recommended Dosage	Per Day
Amino Acids	4GM/kg	_____ GM
Dextrose	1.5GM/kg	_____ GM
Lipids	1GM/kg	_____ GM

Additives (available stock):		Per Dose	Per Dose
KCl	(40mEq/50ml)	_____ mEq	_____ ml
NaAcetate	(40mEq/ml)	_____ mEq	_____ ml
CaGluconate	(45mEq/ml)	_____ mEq	_____ ml
$MgSO_4$	(5mEq/2.5ml)	_____ mEq	_____ ml
Multivit Conc.	———	_____ ml	_____ ml
Zn	(1mg/ml)	_____ mg	_____ ml
Cu	(0.4mg/ml)	_____ mg	_____ ml
Mn	(4mg/3ml)	_____ mg	_____ ml
Cr	(4mcg/ml)	_____ mg	_____ ml
Insulin		_____ U	_____ ml

STANDARD PHARMACY ORDERS:
Always compound TPN / IV using aseptic technique

Pharmacy Technician Name: _____

Pharmacy Technician Signature: _____

Date: _____

ADVENTURE HOSPITAL
TPN PHARMACY ORDER

Patient Name _____

Allergies _____

MR # _____

Calculate the amount of grams needed per day for the standard formula; calculate the ml to be given per liter for the additives. Complete one TPN pharmacy order for each day per patient

Indication for TPN: _____ Wt: _____

Route: ☐ Central Line (CL) ☐ Peripheral Line (PL)

Date: _____

Flow Rate _____ ml/hr, Total ml/day _____, Total L/day _____

Standard Formula:	Recommended Dosage	Per Day
Amino Acids	4GM/kg	_____ GM
Dextrose	1.5GM/kg	_____ GM
Lipids	1GM/kg	_____ GM

Additives (available stock):		Per Dose	Per Dose
KCl	(40mEq/50ml)	_____ mEq	_____ ml
NaAcetate	(40mEq/ml)	_____ mEq	_____ ml
CaGluconate	(45mEq/ml)	_____ mEq	_____ ml
$MgSO_4$	(5mEq/2.5ml)	_____ mEq	_____ ml
Multivit Conc.	———	_____ ml	_____ ml
Zn	(1mg/ml)	_____ mg	_____ ml
Cu	(0.4mg/ml)	_____ mg	_____ ml
Mn	(4mg/3ml)	_____ mg	_____ ml
Cr	(4mcg/ml)	_____ mg	_____ ml
Insulin		_____ U	_____ ml

STANDARD PHARMACY ORDERS:
Always compound TPN / IV using aseptic technique

Pharmacy Technician Name: _____

Pharmacy Technician Signature: _____

Date: _____

ADVENTURE HOSPITAL
TPN PHARMACY ORDER

Patient Name _____

Allergies _____

MR # _____

Calculate the amount of grams needed per day for the standard formula; calculate the ml to be given per liter for the additives. Complete one TPN pharmacy order for each day per patient

Indication for TPN: _____ Wt: _____

Route: ☐ Central Line (CL) ☐ Peripheral Line (PL)

Date: _____

Flow Rate _____ ml/hr, Total ml/day _____, Total L/day _____

Standard Formula:	Recommended Dosage	Per Day
Amino Acids	4GM/kg	_____ GM
Dextrose	1.5GM/kg	_____ GM
Lipids	1GM/kg	_____ GM

Additives (available stock):		Per Dose	Per Dose
KCl	(40mEq/50ml)	_____ mEq	_____ ml
NaAcetate	(40mEq/ml)	_____ mEq	_____ ml
CaGluconate	(45mEq/ml)	_____ mEq	_____ ml
MgSO$_4$	(5mEq/2.5ml)	_____ mEq	_____ ml
Multivit Conc.	_____	_____ ml	_____ ml
Zn	(1mg/ml)	_____ mg	_____ ml
Cu	(0.4mg/ml)	_____ mg	_____ ml
Mn	(4mg/3ml)	_____ mg	_____ ml
Cr	(4mcg/ml)	_____ mg	_____ ml
Insulin		_____ U	_____ ml

STANDARD PHARMACY ORDERS:
Always compound TPN / IV using aseptic technique

Pharmacy Technician Name: _____

Pharmacy Technician Signature: _____

Date: _____

ADVENTURE HOSPITAL
TPN PHARMACY ORDER

Patient Name _____

Allergies _____

MR # _____

Calculate the amount of grams needed per day for the standard formula; calculate the ml to be given per liter for the additives. Complete one TPN pharmacy order for each day per patient

Indication for TPN: _____ Wt: _____

Route: ☐ Central Line (CL) ☐ Peripheral Line (PL)

Date: _____

Flow Rate _____ ml/hr, Total ml/day _____, Total L/day _____

Standard Formula:	Recommended Dosage	Per Day
Amino Acids	4GM/kg	_____ GM
Dextrose	1.5GM/kg	_____ GM
Lipids	1GM/kg	_____ GM

Additives (available stock):		Per Dose	Per Dose
KCl	(40mEq/50ml)	_____ mEq	_____ ml
NaAcetate	(40mEq/ml)	_____ mEq	_____ ml
CaGluconate	(45mEq/ml)	_____ mEq	_____ ml
$MgSO_4$	(5mEq/2.5ml)	_____ mEq	_____ ml
Multivit Conc.	———	_____ ml	_____ ml
Zn	(1mg/ml)	_____ mg	_____ ml
Cu	(0.4mg/ml)	_____ mg	_____ ml
Mn	(4mg/3ml)	_____ mg	_____ ml
Cr	(4mcg/ml)	_____ mg	_____ ml
Insulin		_____ U	_____ ml

STANDARD PHARMACY ORDERS:
Always compound TPN / IV using aseptic technique

Pharmacy Technician Name: _____

Pharmacy Technician Signature: _____

Date: _____

ADVENTURE HOSPITAL
TPN PHARMACY ORDER

Patient Name _____

Allergies _____

MR # _____

Calcuate the amount of grams needed per day for the standard formula; calculate the ml to be given per liter for the additives. Complete one TPN pharmacy order for each day per patient

Indication for TPN: _____ Wt: _____

Route:　☐ Central Line (CL)　☐ Peripheral Line (PL)

Date: _____

Flow Rate _____ ml/hr, Total ml/day _____, Total L/day _____

Standard Formula:	Recommended Dosage	Per Day
Amino Acids	4GM/kg	_____ GM
Dextrose	1.5GM/kg	_____ GM
Lipids	1GM/kg	_____ GM

Additives (available stock):		Per Dose	Per Dose
KCl	(40mEq/50ml)	_____ mEq	_____ ml
NaAcetate	(40mEq/ml)	_____ mEq	_____ ml
CaGluconate	(45mEq/ml)	_____ mEq	_____ ml
$MgSO_4$	(5mEq/2.5ml)	_____ mEq	_____ ml
Multivit Conc.	———	_____ ml	_____ ml
Zn	(1mg/ml)	_____ mg	_____ ml
Cu	(0.4mg/ml)	_____ mg	_____ ml
Mn	(4mg/3ml)	_____ mg	_____ ml
Cr	(4mcg/ml)	_____ mg	_____ ml
Insulin		_____ U	_____ ml

STANDARD PHARMACY ORDERS:
Always compound TPN / IV using aseptic technique

Pharmacy Technician Name: _____

Pharmacy Technician Signature: _____

Date: _____

ADVENTURE HOSPITAL
TPN PHARMACY ORDER

Patient Name _____

Allergies _____

MR # _____

Calculate the amount of grams needed per day for the standard formula; calculate the ml to be given per liter for the additives. Complete one TPN pharmacy order for each day per patient

Indication for TPN: _____ Wt: _____

Route: ☐ Central Line (CL)   ☐ Peripheral Line (PL)

Date: _____

Flow Rate _____ ml/hr, Total ml/day _____, Total L/day _____

Standard Formula:	Recommended Dosage	Per Day
Amino Acids	4GM/kg	_____ GM
Dextrose	1.5GM/kg	_____ GM
Lipids	1GM/kg	_____ GM

Additives (available stock):		Per Dose	Per Dose
KCl	(40mEq/50ml)	_____ mEq	_____ ml
NaAcetate	(40mEq/ml)	_____ mEq	_____ ml
CaGluconate	(45mEq/ml)	_____ mEq	_____ ml
$MgSO_4$	(5mEq/2.5ml)	_____ mEq	_____ ml
Multivit Conc.	———	_____ ml	_____ ml
Zn	(1mg/ml)	_____ mg	_____ ml
Cu	(0.4mg/ml)	_____ mg	_____ ml
Mn	(4mg/3ml)	_____ mg	_____ ml
Cr	(4mcg/ml)	_____ mg	_____ ml
Insulin		_____ U	_____ ml

STANDARD PHARMACY ORDERS:
Always compound TPN / IV using aseptic technique

Pharmacy Technician Name: _____

Pharmacy Technician Signature: _____

Date: _____

ADVENTURE HOSPITAL
TPN PHARMACY ORDER

Patient Name _____

Allergies _____

MR # _____

Calculate the amount of grams needed per day for the standard formula; calculate the ml to be given per liter for the additives. Complete one TPN pharmacy order for each day per patient

Indication for TPN: _____ Wt: _____

Route: ☐ Central Line (CL)   ☐ Peripheral Line (PL)

Date: _____

Flow Rate _____ ml/hr, Total ml/day _____, Total L/day _____

Standard Formula:	Recommended Dosage	Per Day
Amino Acids	4GM/kg	_____ GM
Dextrose	1.5GM/kg	_____ GM
Lipids	1GM/kg	_____ GM

Additives (available stock):		Per Dose	Per Dose
KCl	(40mEq/50ml)	_____ mEq	_____ ml
NaAcetate	(40mEq/ml)	_____ mEq	_____ ml
CaGluconate	(45mEq/ml)	_____ mEq	_____ ml
MgSO$_4$	(5mEq/2.5ml)	_____ mEq	_____ ml
Multivit Conc.	———	_____ ml	_____ ml
Zn	(1mg/ml)	_____ mg	_____ ml
Cu	(0.4mg/ml)	_____ mg	_____ ml
Mn	(4mg/3ml)	_____ mg	_____ ml
Cr	(4mcg/ml)	_____ mg	_____ ml
Insulin		_____ U	_____ ml

STANDARD PHARMACY ORDERS:
Always compound TPN / IV using aseptic technique

Pharmacy Technician Name: _____

Pharmacy Technician Signature: _____

Date: _____

ADVENTURE HOSPITAL
TPN PHARMACY ORDER

Patient Name _____

Allergies _____

MR # _____

Calculate the amount of grams needed per day for the standard formula; calculate the ml to be given per liter for the additives. Complete one TPN pharmacy order for each day per patient

Indication for TPN: _____ Wt: _____

Route: ☐ Central Line (CL)   ☐ Peripheral Line (PL)

Date: _____

Flow Rate _____ ml/hr, Total ml/day _____, Total L/day _____

Standard Formula:		Recommended Dosage	Per Day
Amino Acids		4GM/kg	_____ GM
Dextrose		1.5GM/kg	_____ GM
Lipids		1GM/kg	_____ GM

Additives (available stock):		Per Dose	Per Dose
KCl	(40mEq/50ml)	_____ mEq	_____ ml
NaAcetate	(40mEq/ml)	_____ mEq	_____ ml
CaGluconate	(45mEq/ml)	_____ mEq	_____ ml
MgSO$_4$	(5mEq/2.5ml)	_____ mEq	_____ ml
Multivit Conc.	────	_____ ml	_____ ml
Zn	(1mg/ml)	_____ mg	_____ ml
Cu	(0.4mg/ml)	_____ mg	_____ ml
Mn	(4mg/3ml)	_____ mg	_____ ml
Cr	(4mcg/ml)	_____ mg	_____ ml
Insulin		_____ U	_____ ml

STANDARD PHARMACY ORDERS:
Always compound TPN / IV using aseptic technique

Pharmacy Technician Name: _____

Pharmacy Technician Signature: _____

Date: _____

Lab 20: Billing

OBJECTIVE

The student will learn how to read difficult insurance cards and how to read a formulary.

EXERCISE 1

1. Using the Bansal Formulary (page 198), look up the following prescriptions.

2. Write the brand name of the medication and classification (class).

3. Using the provided insurance cards (page 188), provide the copay amount.

4. Provide any restrictions for the medication by using the formulary.

5. Fill out the TAR form (page 193) for all prescriptions that need a medical justification or that are not on the formulary. Additional TAR forms can be found in the Appendix.

Dr. Phull, H	Dr. Diver, Skye	Dr. Bansal, S	Dr. Perez, C
Dr. Mundian, K	Dr. Virdee, S	Dr. Climber, R	Dr. Racer, C
Dr. Dhillon, S	Dr. Chana, C	Dr. McDonald, R	Dr. Radia, K

Bansal Urgent Care

Name: *Jack Smith*   Date: _____
Address: _____
RX

     Folic Acid 1mg
         1 qd X 3months

DAW ☐   Refill ⑫   MD *Radia, K.*   Lic. No : _____
                 DEA#

Dr. Phull, H	Dr. Diver, Skye	Dr. Bansal, S	Dr. Perez, C
Dr. Mundian, K	Dr. Virdee, S	Dr. Climber, R	Dr. Racer, C
Dr. Dhillon, S	Dr. Chana, C	Dr. McDonald, R	Dr. Radia, K

Bansal Urgent Care

Name: *Oliver Daniel*   Date: _____
Address: _____
RX

     Abacavir Sulfate 300mg #120
         Tqid

DAW ☐   Refill ⑫   MD *Racer, C*   Lic. No : _____
                 DEA#

Dr. Phull, H   Dr. Diver, Skye   Dr. Bansal, S   Dr. Perez, C
Dr. Mundian, K   Dr. Virdee, S   Dr. Climber, R   Dr. Racer, C
Dr. Dhillon, S   Dr. Chana, C   Dr. McDonald, R   Dr. Radia, K

Bansal Urgent Care

Name: _Gyn Derella_____ Date: _____
Address: _____
RX

    Ativan 2mg   #30
         T qd prn anxiety

DAW ☒   Refill _Ø_   MD _Bansal_   Lic. No :
                       DEA#

Dr. Phull, H   Dr. Diver, Skye   Dr. Bansal, S   Dr. Perez, C
Dr. Mundian, K   Dr. Virdee, S   Dr. Climber, R   Dr. Racer, C
Dr. Dhillon, S   Dr. Chana, C   Dr. McDonald, R   Dr. Radia, K

Bansal Urgent Care

Name: _Lolly Pop_____ Date: _____
Address: _____
RX

    Carbachol 1.5% #15mls
      T-TT gtt into each eye x 10d.
             everyday

DAW ☐   Refill _Ø_   MD _Climber, R._   Lic. No :
                       DEA#

Dr. Phull, H   Dr. Diver, Skye   Dr. Bansal, S   Dr. Perez, C
Dr. Mundian, K   Dr. Virdee, S   Dr. Climber, R   Dr. Racer, C
Dr. Dhillon, S   Dr. Chana, C   Dr. McDonald, R   Dr. Radia, K

Bansal Urgent Care

Name: _John Wayne_____ Date: _____
Address: _____
RX

    Cephalexin 500mg #21
          T tid x 7d

DAW ☐   Refill _Ø_   MD _Chana, C_   Lic. No :
                       DEA#

Dr. Phull, H   Dr. Diver, Skye   Dr. Bansal, S   Dr. Perez, C
Dr. Mundian, K   Dr. Virdee, S   Dr. Climber, R   Dr. Racer, C
Dr. Dhillon, S   Dr. Chana, C   Dr. McDonald, R   Dr. Radia, K

Bansal Urgent Care

Name: _Chris Columbus_____ Date: _9 yrs old_
Address: _____
RX

    Cetixime 100mg/5ml #50ml
        T tsp qd x 10d.

DAW ☐   Refill _Ø_   MD _Diver, Skye_   Lic. No :
                       DEA#

Dr. Phull, H   Dr. Diver, Skye   Dr. Bansal, S   Dr. Perez, C
Dr. Mundian, K   Dr. Virdee, S   Dr. Climber, R   Dr. Racer, C
Dr. Dhillon, S   Dr. Chana, C   Dr. McDonald, R   Dr. Radia, K

Bansal Urgent Care

Name: _Alex Keaton_____ Date: _____
Address: _____
RX

    Codeine/ APAP #3   #45
        T-TT q4-6hrs prn severe pain

DAW ☐   Refill _Ø_   MD _Virdee, S_   Lic. No :
                       DEA#

Dr. Phull, H   Dr. Diver, Skye   Dr. Bansal, S   Dr. Perez, C
Dr. Mundian, K   Dr. Virdee, S   Dr. Climber, R   Dr. Racer, C
Dr. Dhillon, S   Dr. Chana, C   Dr. McDonald, R   Dr. Radia, K

Bansal Urgent Care

Name: _Decimal Dewey_____ Date: _____
Address: _____
RX

    Delaviridine Mesylate 200mg
         T qd x 30d

DAW ☐   Refill _____   MD _____   Lic. No :
                       DEA#

Dr. Phull, H   Dr. Diver, Skye   Dr. Bansal, S   Dr. Perez, C
Dr. Mundian, K   Dr. Virdee, S   Dr. Climber, R   Dr. Racer, C
Dr. Dhillon, S   Dr. Chana, C   Dr. McDonald, R   Dr. Radia, K

Bansal Urgent Care

Name: _Prop Agand_____ Date: _____
Address: _____
RX

    Meclizine Hydrochloride 25mg
      chew/swallow T tab qd prn dizziness

DAW ☐   Refill _②_   MD _Phull, H._   Lic. No :
                       DEA#

Dr. Phull, H   Dr. Diver, Skye   Dr. Bansal, S   Dr. Perez, C
Dr. Mundian, K   Dr. Virdee, S   Dr. Climber, R   Dr. Racer, C
Dr. Dhillon, S   Dr. Chana, C   Dr. McDonald, R   Dr. Radia, K

Bansal Urgent Care

Name: _Achilles Heel_____ Date: _____
Address: _____
RX

    thiothixene 20mg   #30
         T qd x 30d

DAW ☐   Refill _②_   MD _Dhillon, S_   Lic. No :
                       DEA#

Dr. Phull, H	Dr. Diver, Skye	Dr. Bansal, S	Dr. Perez, C
Dr. Mundian, K	Dr. Virdee, S	Dr. Climber, R	Dr. Racer, C
Dr. Dhillon, S	Dr. Chana, C	Dr. McDonald, R	Dr. Radia, K

Bansal Urgent Care

Name: Aditya Singh   Date: _____
Address: _____
RX

Omeprazole 20mg   #60
i-ii q12hr prn GERD

DAW ☐   Refill Ø   MD Mundian, K.   Lic. No : _____
DEA# _____

Dr. Phull, H	Dr. Diver, Skye	Dr. Bansal, S	Dr. Perez, C
Dr. Mundian, K	Dr. Virdee, S	Dr. Climber, R	Dr. Racer, C
Dr. Dhillon, S	Dr. Chana, C	Dr. McDonald, R	Dr. Radia, K

Bansal Urgent Care

Name: Aeron Welsh   Date: _____
Address: _____
RX

Paroxetine 40mg   #30
i qam

DAW ☐   Refill ②   MD S Bansal   Lic. No : _____
DEA# _____

Dr. Phull, H	Dr. Diver, Skye	Dr. Bansal, S	Dr. Perez, C
Dr. Mundian, K	Dr. Virdee, S	Dr. Climber, R	Dr. Racer, C
Dr. Dhillon, S	Dr. Chana, C	Dr. McDonald, R	Dr. Radia, K

Bansal Urgent Care

Name: Devon Bansal   Date: _____
Address: _____
RX

Temazepam   7.5mg   #30
i qhs x 30d

DAW ☐   Refill Ø   MD McDonald, R   Lic. No : _____
DEA# _____

Dr. Phull, H	Dr. Diver, Skye	Dr. Bansal, S	Dr. Perez, C
Dr. Mundian, K	Dr. Virdee, S	Dr. Climber, R	Dr. Racer, C
Dr. Dhillon, S	Dr. Chana, C	Dr. McDonald, R	Dr. Radia, K

Bansal Urgent Care

Name: Chris Chana   Date: _____
Address: _____
RX

Tazarotene Gel 0.05% #30g
apply sparing to affected skin

DAW ☐   Refill ②   MD S Bansal   Lic. No : _____
DEA# _____

Dr. Phull, H	Dr. Diver, Skye	Dr. Bansal, S	Dr. Perez, C
Dr. Mundian, K	Dr. Virdee, S	Dr. Climber, R	Dr. Racer, C
Dr. Dhillon, S	Dr. Chana, C	Dr. McDonald, R	Dr. Radia, K

Bansal Urgent Care

Name: Kim Mundian   Date: _____
Address: _____
RX

Benazpril HCL/HCTZ ⑩   #30
i qd x 30d (↑BP)

DAW ☐   Refill ②   MD S Bansal   Lic. No : _____
DEA# _____

Dr. Phull, H	Dr. Diver, Skye	Dr. Bansal, S	Dr. Perez, C
Dr. Mundian, K	Dr. Virdee, S	Dr. Climber, R	Dr. Racer, C
Dr. Dhillon, S	Dr. Chana, C	Dr. McDonald, R	Dr. Radia, K

Bansal Urgent Care

Name: Raj Dhillon   Date: _____
Address: _____
RX

Erythromycin oint 5gms
apply 1"ribbon to
each eye x 7d.

DAW ☐   Refill ②   MD S Bansal   Lic. No : _____
DEA# _____

Dr. Phull, H	Dr. Diver, Skye	Dr. Bansal, S	Dr. Perez, C
Dr. Mundian, K	Dr. Virdee, S	Dr. Climber, R	Dr. Racer, C
Dr. Dhillon, S	Dr. Chana, C	Dr. McDonald, R	Dr. Radia, K

Bansal Urgent Care

Name: Alvis Chipmunk   Date: _____
Address: _____
RX

Zidovudine   50mg/5ml   #150
50mg qd x 30d

DAW ☐   Refill ⑧   MD Perez, Christine   Lic. No : _____
DEA# _____

Dr. Phull, H	Dr. Diver, Skye	Dr. Bansal, S	Dr. Perez, C
Dr. Mundian, K	Dr. Virdee, S	Dr. Climber, R	Dr. Racer, C
Dr. Dhillon, S	Dr. Chana, C	Dr. McDonald, R	Dr. Radia, K

Bansal Urgent Care

Name: Mister Amen   Date: _____
Address: _____
RX

Danocrine   100mg   #360
iv caps qid x 30 months

DAW ☐   Refill Ø   MD S Bansal   Lic. No : _____
DEA# _____

Dr. Phull, H	Dr. Diver, Skye	Dr. Bansal, S	Dr. Perez, C
Dr. Mundian, K	Dr. Virdee, S	Dr. Climber, R	Dr. Racer, C
Dr. Dhillon, S	Dr. Chana, C	Dr. McDonald, R	Dr. Radia, K

Bansal Urgent Care

Name: _Belal Cardea_ Date: _____

Address: _____

RX

Diazepam 10mg #30
Tqd x30d

DAW ☐ Refill ② MD _Radia, K._ Lic. No : _____
DEA# _____

Dr. Phull, H	Dr. Diver, Skye	Dr. Bansal, S	Dr. Perez, C
Dr. Mundian, K	Dr. Virdee, S	Dr. Climber, R	Dr. Racer, C
Dr. Dhillon, S	Dr. Chana, C	Dr. McDonald, R	Dr. Radia, K

Bansal Urgent Care

Name: _Castor Troy_ Date: _____

Address: _____

RX

Sildenafil 50mg #30
T tab 1hr prior to sexual activity.

DAW ☐ Refill ③ MD _Racer, Cas_ Lic. No : _____
DEA# _____

Table 20-1

Patient Name	Brand Name	FormularyDrug? Y or N	Restrictions	Class	Copay Amount
Example: Jack Smith	Folvite	Y	None	Antianemic	$2.00
					$
					$
					$
					$
					$
					$
					$
					$
					$
					$
					$
					$
					$
					$
					$
					$
					$
					$
					$

*All medications that are not on the Bansal Formulary must pay the NF copay.
**Not all medications have restrictions.
***All insurance companies use the Bansal Formulary for this exercise.

Bansal/Perez Insurance

Jack Smith
Group number: **5269854**
ID: **GHUEP**

OV: $5	Dental: $15	ER: $0	Acupuncture: $55
RX: $2	NFRX: $20	Vision: $25	Chiropractor: $3

Compass Insurance

Oliver Daniel

PCC: **Dr. Mundian**
Medical Number: **00235**

ID number: **74G5T89DF**
MD ID: **DFRS41**

HMO

OV: $5	Dental: $15	ER: $0	Acupuncture: $55
RX: $5	NFRX: $20	Vision: $25	Chiropractor: $3

Red Star Insurance

Cyn Derella
Group number: **8569784**
Number: **23584**
Medical ID: **SKB675**

Employee

Dr. Chana, C

OV: $5	Dental: $15	ER: $0	Acupuncture: $55
RX: $2	NFRX: $10	Vision: $25	Chiropractor: $3

Knight Insurance

Lolly Pop
Group number: **ASDWAX**
Member ID: **25698541**

Insurer: **Self**

OV: $5	Dental: $15	ER: $0	Acupuncture: $55
RX: $20	NFRX: $30	Vision: $25	Chiropractor: $3

Knight Insurance

John Wayne
Group number: **555888996**
Physician ID: **87DEFR**

Employer Number: **25896**
Member ID: **148569AB**

| OV: $5 | Dental: $15 | ER: $0 | Acupuncture: $55 |
| RX: $2 | NFRX: $10 | Vision: $25 | Chiropractor: $3 |

Bansal/Perez Insurance

Chris Columbus
Group number: **WECVYTG**
ID: **4521963**

| OV: $5 | Dental: $15 | ER: $0 | Acupuncture: $55 |
| RX: $2 | NFRX: $10 | Vision: $25 | Chiropractor: $3 |

Bansal/Perez Insurance

Alex Keaton
Group number: **7426985**
ID: **LPOFEC**

| OV: $5 | Dental: $15 | ER: $0 | Acupuncture: $55 |
| RX: $10 | NFRX: $60 | Vision: $25 | Chiropractor: $3 |

Pharmacy Insurance

Decimal Dewey
Group number: **E4V8T59F**
ID: **FS26A8D**

Pharmacy ID: **57896**
Member ID: **568-885-5632**
PC: **Dr. Phull**

| OV: $5 | Dental: $15 | ER: $0 | Acupuncture: $55 |
| RX: $26 | NFRX: $30 | Vision: $25 | Chiropractor: $3 |

Bansal/Perez Insurance

Prop Aganda
Group number: **85694**
ID: **GSDV**

| OV: $5 | Dental: $15 | ER: $0 | Acupuncture: $55 |
| RX: $20 | NFRX: $40 | Vision: $25 | Chiropractor: $3 |

Pharmacy Insurance

Achilles Heel   Pharmacy ID: **58654**
Group number: **7891235**
ID: **QWSDGH**

| OV: $5 | Dental: $15 | ER: $0 | Acupuncture: $55 |
| RX: $10 | NFRX: $35 | Vision: $25 | Chiropractor: $3 |

Bansal/Perez Insurance

Aditya Singh
Group number: **7425962**
ID: **FDZFG**

| OV: $5 | Dental: $15 | ER: $0 | Acupuncture: $55 |
| RX: $2 | NFRX: $10 | Vision: $25 | Chiropractor: $3 |

B&D Consulting
Bansal Ins.

Aeron Welsh
Employer: **Self**
Group number: **745962**
Employee ID: **1**
Medical ID: **EWWVH**   PC: **Dr. Bansal**

| OV: $5 | Dental: $15 | ER: $0 | Acupuncture: $55 |
| RX: $15 | NFRX: $70 | Vision: $25 | Chiropractor: $3 |

Navigation Insurance Co.

Devon Bansal   Member ID: **45896**
Dependent: **3**
Group number: **745239**
Pharmacy ID: **SDFSFH**

OV: $5   Dental: $15   ER: $0   Acupuncture: $55
RX: $25   NFRX: $20   Vision: $25   Chiropractor: $3

Urgent Care Insurance

Chris Chana
Group number: **54894541**
ID: **F45F45**

OV: N/A   Dental: N/A   ER: $0   Acupuncture: $55
RX: $20   NFRX: $30   Vision: N/A   Chiropractor: N/A

Mundian and Associates

Kim Mundian
Group number: **755487DF**
ID: **FDFDF8**

OV: $5   Dental: $15   ER: $0   Acupuncture: $55
RX: $12   NFRX: $50   Vision: $25   Chiropractor: $3

Rock Art Insurance

Raj Dhillon   Employer: **Dental Co.**
Group number: **85468DFG**   Employer ID: **58796**
Member ID: **FKEG5861**

OV: $5   Dental: $15   ER: $0   Acupuncture: $55
RX: $0   NFRX: $30   Vision: $25   Chiropractor: $3

Urgent Care Insurance

Alvis Chipmunk
Group number: **78425F**
Billing ID: **FDBDS**

| OV: $5 | Dental: $15 | ER: $0 | Acupuncture: $55 |
| RX: $6 | NFRX: $8 | Vision: $25 | Chiropractor: $3 |

Bansal/Perez Insurance

Mister Amen
Group number: **859632**
ID: **FDGFD**

| OV: $5 | Dental: $15 | ER: $0 | Acupuncture: $55 |
| RX: $25 | NFRX: $80 | Vision: $44 | Chiropractor: $3 |

Adventure Insurance

Belal Cardea   Medical ID: **789654**
Group number: **859671**   PCC: **Dr. Diver, S**
Member ID: **FDSDF**

| OV: $8 | Dental: $15 | ER: $0 | Acupuncture: $55 |
| RX: $2 | NFRX: $5 | Vision: $25 | Chiropractor: $3 |

Climbing Insurance

Castor Troy   PCC: **Dr. Climber, Rok**
Group number: **742814**   PCC ID: **5893214**
Billing ID: **FDSGFB**

| OV: $5 | Dental: $15 | ER: $0 | Acupuncture: $55 |
| RX: $2 | NFRX: $10 | Vision: $25 | Chiropractor: $3 |

Authorization for Treatment

Patient Name _____
 Last   First   Middle

Mailing Address _____

Subscriber ID_____ Patient Date of Birth _____

Sex M F   Relationship to subscriber _____

Subscriber Phone Number _____

Description of Diagnosis _____

Medical Justification:

_____

_____

_____

Drug Name and Strength	Directions	Quantity / Charge	NDC #	Initials of Provider / Title

Name of Pharmacy _____

Address_____

Phone Number _____

Provider Signature _____ Date_____

Authorization for Treatment

Patient Name _____

                               Last   First   Middle

Mailing Address _____

Subscriber ID_____ Patient Date of Birth _____

Sex   M   F   Relationship to subscriber _____

Subscriber Phone Number _____

Description of Diagnosis _____

Medical Justification:

_____

_____

_____

Drug Name and Strength	Directions	Quantity / Charge	NDC #	Initials of Provider / Title

Name of Pharmacy_____

Address_____

Phone Number _____

Provider Signature _____ Date_____

Authorization for Treatment

Patient Name _____

                      Last   First   Middle

Mailing Address _____

Subscriber ID_____ Patient Date of Birth _____

Sex   M   F   Relationship to subscriber _____

Subscriber Phone Number _____

Description of Diagnosis _____

Medical Justification:

_____

_____

_____

Drug Name and Strength	Directions	Quantity / Charge	NDC #	Initials of Provider / Title

Name of Pharmacy_____

Address_____

Phone Number _____

Provider Signature _____ Date_____

Authorization for Treatment

Patient Name _____

                            Last   First   Middle

Mailing Address _____

Subscriber ID_____ Patient Date of Birth _____

Sex M   F   Relationship to subscriber _____

Subscriber Phone Number _____

Description of Diagnosis _____

Medical Justification:

_____

_____

_____

Drug Name and Strength	Directions	Quantity / Charge	NDC #	Initials of Provider / Title

Name of Pharmacy_____

Address_____

Phone Number _____

Provider Signature _____ Date_____

Authorization for Treatment

Patient Name _____

                   Last   First   Middle

Mailing Address _____

Subscriber ID_____ Patient Date of Birth _____

Sex M F   Relationship to subscriber _____

Subscriber Phone Number _____

Description of Diagnosis _____

Medical Justification:

_____

_____

_____

Drug Name and Strength	Directions	Quantity / Charge	NDC #	Initials of Provider / Title

Name of Pharmacy_____

Address_____

Phone Number _____

Provider Signature _____ Date_____

BANSAL FORMULARY* ───

Abacavir Sulfate

Tablets	300mg	
Liquid	20mg/cc	

Restricted to use as combination therapy in the treatment of Human Immunodeficiency Virus (HIV) infection.

Abacavir Sulfate and Lamivudine

Tablets	600mg/300mg	ea

Restricted to use as combination therapy in the treatment of Human Immunodeficiency Virus (HIV) infection.

Abacavir Sulfate, Lamivudine, and Zidovudine

Tablets	300mg/150mg/300mg	ea

Restricted to use alone or as combination therapy in the treatment of Human Immunodeficiency Virus (HIV) infection.

Acebutolol

Capsules	200mg	ea
	400mg	ea

Acetazolamide

Tablets	125mg	ea
	250mg	ea
Capsules, sustained release	500mg	ea

Acetic Acid

Irrigating solution	0.25%	250 cc	cc
		500 cc	cc

Acetic Acid with Aluminum Acetate

Otic solution	2%	cc

Acetic Acid with Hydrocortisone

Otic solution

─────────────

*The formulary is a sample obtained from the Medi-cal system. This can be viewed at www.medi-cal.ca.gov.

Acyclovir

Capsules	200mg		ea
Tablets	400mg		ea
	800mg		ea

Restricted to use in patients with herpes genitalis, immunocompromised patients and patients with herpes zoster (shingles).

Albuterol

Inhaler with adapter	17Gm		Gm
Inhaler without adapter	17Gm		Gm

Albuterol Sulfate

Tablets or capsules	2mg		ea
	4mg		ea

Amoxicillin Trihydrate

Solution or suspension	125mg/5 cc	80 cc	cc
		100 cc	cc
		150 cc	cc
	250mg/5 cc	80 cc	cc
		100 cc	cc
		150 cc	cc
		200 cc	cc
Pediatric drops	50mg/cc	15 cc	cc
		30 cc	cc
Capsules	250mg		ea
	500mg		ea
Chewable tablets	250mg		ea

Atenolol

Tablets	25mg		ea
	50mg		ea
	100mg		ea

Atorvastatin Calcium

Tablets	10mg		ea
	20mg		ea
	40mg		ea
	80mg		ea

Azithromycin

Tablets	250mg		ea

Restricted to a maximum quantity per dispensing of eight (8) tablets and a maximum of two (2) dispensings in any 30-day period.

Tablets	500mg		ea

Restricted to a maximum quantity per dispensing of four (4) tablets and a maximum of two (2) dispensings in any 30-day period.

Tablets	600mg		ea

Restricted to use in the prevention of infections caused by Mycobacterium organisms.

Powder packet	1Gm		ea
Suspension	100mg/5 cc	15 cc	cc
	200mg/5 cc	15 cc	cc
		22.5 cc	cc

Baclofen

Tablets or capsules	10mg		ea
	20mg		ea

Benazepril HCL

Tablets	5mg		ea
	10mg		ea
	20mg		ea
	40mg		ea

Benazepril HCL and Hydrochlorothiazide

Tablets	5mg–6.25mg		ea
	10mg–12.5mg		ea
	20mg–12.5mg		ea
	20mg–25mg		ea

Benzoyl Peroxide

Gel	5%		Gm
	10%		Gm

Benztropine Mesylate

Injection	1mg/cc	2 cc	cc
Tablets	0.5mg		ea
	1mg		ea
	2mg		ea

Carbachol

Ophthalmic	0.75%	15 cc	cc
		30 cc	cc
	1.5%	15 cc	cc

Carbamazepine

Capsules, extended release	200mg		ea
	300mg		ea
Chewable tablets	100mg		ea

Carbenicillin

Tablets	382mg		ea

Carbidopa and Levodopa

Tablets	10mg/100mg		ea
	25mg/100mg		ea

Carvedilol

Tablets	3.125mg		ea
	6.25mg		ea

Restricted to use for the treatment of mild to severe heart failure.

Cefixime

Liquid	100mg/5 cc	50 cc	cc
		75 cc	cc
		100 cc	cc

Restricted to use for individuals less than 8 years old with otitis media infections.

Tablets	400mg		ea

Restricted to use in the treatment of Neisseria gonorrhoeae, and to a maximum quantity per dispensing of one (1) tablet and a maximum of one (1) dispensing in any 30-day period.

Cephalexin

Capsules	250mg		ea
	500mg		ea
Solution or suspension	125mg/5 cc	100 cc	cc
		200 cc	cc
	250mg/5 cc	100 cc	cc
		200 cc	cc

Cinacalcet HCL

Tablets	30mg		ea
	60mg		ea
	90mg		ea

Restricted to use in secondary hyperparathyroidism in patients with chronic kidney disease on dialysis or hypercalcemia in patients with parathyroid carcinoma.

Ciprofloxacin

Suspension, oral	5%		cc
	10%		cc

Restricted to use in the treatment of (1) lower respiratory tract infections in persons aged 50 years and older; (2) osteomyelitis; and (3) pulmonary exacerbation of cystic fibrosis.

Ciprofloxacin and Ciprofloxacin HCL

Tablets, extended release	500mg		ea

Restricted to use in the treatment of urinary tract infections and to a maximum of three (3) tablets per dispensing and a maximum of two (2) dispensings in any 30-day period.

Tablets, extended release	1000mg		ea

Restricted to use in the treatment of urinary tract infections, including pyelonephritis and to a maximum of ten (10) tablets per dispensing and a maximum of two (2) dispensings in any 30-day period.

Clarithromycin

Tablets, extended release	500mg		ea
Tablets	250mg		ea
	500mg		ea

Restricted to use in the prevention and treatment of infections caused by Mycobacterium organisms and in the treatment of active duodenal ulcer associated with Helicobacter pylori.

Liquid	125mg/5 cc		cc
	250mg/5 cc		cc

Restricted to use in the prevention and treatment of infections caused by Mycobacterium organisms and in the treatment of active duodenal ulcer associated with Helicobacter pylori

Clindamycin Hydrochloride

Tablets or capsules	75mg		ea
	150mg		ea
	300mg		ea

Clindamycin Phosphate

Injection	150mg/cc	2 cc	cc
		4 cc	cc
		6 cc	cc
		60 cc	cc
Vaginal cream	2%	5.8 Gm	Gm
Vaginal cream	2%	40 Gm	Gm

Clonazepam

Tablets	0.5mg		ea
	1.0mg		ea
	2.0mg		ea

Restricted to therapy lasting up to 90 days from the dispensing date of the first prescription.

Codeine and Acetaminophen

Tablets or capsules	15mg–300 to 325mg		ea

Restricted to a maximum dispensing quantity of 60 tablets or capsules and a maximum of three (3) dispensings in any 75-day period.

	30mg–300 to 325mg		ea

Restricted to a maximum dispensing quantity of 45 tablets or capsules and a maximum of three (3) dispensings in any 75-day period.

Liquid	12mg–120mg/5 cc		cc

Codeine and Aspirin

Tablets or capsules	15mg–325mg		ea

Restricted to a maximum dispensing quantity of 60 tablets or capsules and a maximum of three (3) dispensings in any 75-day period.

	30mg–325mg		ea

Restricted to a maximum dispensing quantity of 45 tablets or capsules and a maximum of three (3) dispensings in any 75-day period.

Codeine Phosphate

Injection	30mg/cc	1 cc	cc
	60mg/cc	1 cc	cc

Delaviridine Mesylate

Tablets	100mg		ea
	200mg		ea

Restricted to use as combination therapy in the treatment of Human Immunodeficiency Virus (HIV) infection.

Dexamethasone

Elixir	0.5mg/5 cc	100 cc	cc
Tablets			ea
Injection	4mg/cc	5 cc	cc
		10 cc	cc
Ophthalmic ointment	0.05%		Gm

Diazepam

Injection	5mg/cc	2 cc	cc
	5mg/cc	10 cc	cc
Tablets	2mg	500's	ea
	5mg	500's	ea
	10mg	500's	ea

Restricted to use in cerebral palsy, athetoid states, or spinal cord degeneration.

Diclofenac Sodium

Ophthalmic solution	0.1%	cc
Tablets	25mg	ea
	50mg	ea
	75mg	ea

Restricted to use for arthritis.

Diflunisal

Tablets or capsules	250mg	ea
	500mg	ea

Restricted to use for arthritis.

Donepezil HCL

Restricted to treatment of mild to moderate dementia of the Alzheimer's type.

Tablets or orally disintegrating tablets	5mg	ea
	10mg	ea

Doxycycline Hyclate

Tablets or capsules	20mg		ea

Restricted to use as an adjunct therapy to scaling and root planing in patients with adult periondontitis and to a maximum quantity of 60 capsules per dispensing and a maximum of nine (9) dispensings in any 12-month period.

Capsules	50mg		ea
	100mg		ea
Tablets	100mg		ea

Erythromycin

Ophthalmic ointment			Gm
Topical solution 2%	60 cc		cc

Erythromycin and Sulfisoxazole

Liquid	200mg–600mg/5 cc	100 cc	cc
		150 cc	cc
		200 cc	cc

Erythromycin Base

Tablets	250mg		ea
	500mg		ea
Tablets, delayed release	333mg		ea
Capsules, delayed release	250mg		ea

Estradiol

Tablets	0.5mg		ea
	1mg		ea
	2mg		ea
Transdermal system once-weekly patch	0.025mg		ea
	0.05mg		ea
	0.075mg		ea

Fluvastatin Sodium

Capsules	20mg		ea
	40mg		ea
Tablets, extended release	80mg		ea

Fluvastatin Maleate

Tablets	25mg		ea
	50mg		ea
	100mg		ea

Folic Acid

Tablets	1mg		ea

Formoterol Fumarate

Capsules for oral inhalation	12mcg		ea

Fosamprenavir Calcium

Restricted to use as a combination therapy in the treatment of Human Immunodeficiency Virus (HIV) infection.

Tablets	700mg		ea
Oral Suspension	50mg/cc		cc

Foscarnet Sodium

Injection	24mg/cc	250 cc	cc
		500 cc	cc

Restricted to use in patients with AIDS or AIDS-related conditions.

Furosemide

Injection	10mg/cc		cc
Tablets	20mg		ea
	40mg	500s	ea
	80mg		ea
Liquid	10mg/cc	60 cc	cc
		120 cc	cc

Galantamine Hydrobromide

Tablets	4mg		ea
	8mg		ea
	12mg		ea
Extended-release capsules	8mg		ea
	16mg		ea
	24mg		ea

Restricted to treatment of mild to moderate dementia of the Alzheimer's type.

Ganciclovir

Capsules	250mg		ea
	500mg		ea

Restricted to use in the treatment of AIDS-related conditions.

Ganciclovir Sodium

Powder for injection	500mg/vial		ea

Restricted to use in the treatment of AIDS-related conditions.

Gentamicin

Ophthalmic ointment	0.3%		Gm
Ophthalmic solution/drops	0.3%	5 cc	cc
		15 cc	cc

Loxapine HCL

Solution	25mg/cc		cc
Injection	50mg/cc		cc

Loxapine Succinate

Capsules	5mg		ea
	10mg		ea

Mebendazole

Tablets, chewable	100mg		ea

Meclizine Hydrochloride

Tablets	25mg		ea
Tablets, chewable	25mg		ea

Naproxen

Tablets or capsules	250mg		ea
	375mg		ea
	500mg		ea
Liquid	125mg	5 cc	cc

Natamycin

Ophthalmic suspension	5%	15 cc	cc

Nateglinide

Tablets	60mg		ea
	120mg		ea

Nelfinavir Mesylate

Tablets	250mg		ea
	625mg		ea
Oral powder	50mg/Gm		Gm

Restricted to use as combination therapy in the treatment of Human Immunodeficiency Virus (HIV) infection.

Neomycin

Tablets	0.5Gm		ea
Liquid	125mg/5 cc		cc

Ofloxacin

Ophthalmic solution	0.3%		cc
Otic solution	0.3%	5 cc	cc
	10 cc		cc
Tablets	200mg		ea
	300mg		ea

Restricted to use in the treatment of sexually transmitted diseases.

Ondansetron

Injection	2mg/cc	cc

Restricted to a maximum of 32 mg per dispensing.

Tablets	4mg	ea
	8mg	ea
Tablets, orally disintegrating	4mg	ea
	8mg	ea

Restricted to a maximum of 12 tablets per dispensing.

Oxycodone and Acetaminophen

Tablets or capsules	5mg–500mg	ea
	5mg–325mg	ea

Oxycodone HCL

Tablets or capsules	5mg	ea
	15mg	ea
	30mg	ea

Restricted to a maximum of 90 tablets or capsules per dispensing and a maximum of three dispensings of any strength in a 75-day period. Exceptions to this restriction require prior authorization.

Tablets, controlled release	10mg	ea
	20mg	ea
	40mg	ea
	80mg	ea
	160mg	ea

Restricted to a maximum of 90 tablets per dispensing and a maximum of three dispensings of any strength in a 75-day period. Exceptions to this restriction require prior authorization.

Solution		cc
Concentrate		cc

Paroxetine Mesylate

Tablets	10mg		ea
	20mg		ea
	30mg		ea
	40mg		ea

Penicillin V (K)

Tablets	125mg		ea
	250mg		ea
	500mg		ea
Liquid	125mg/5 cc	100 cc	cc
		150 cc	cc
		200 cc	cc
	250mg/5 cc	100 cc	cc
		150 cc	cc
		200 cc	cc

Ribavirin

Capsules	200mg		ea
Tablets	200mg		ea

Restricted to use as combination therapy in the treatment of Hepatitis C. Also restricted to therapy lasting up to 48 weeks from the dispensing date of the first prescription.

Rifabutin

Capsules	150mg		ea

Restricted to use in the prevention of disseminated Mycobacterium Avium Complex (MAC) disease in patients with advanced HIV infection.

Rifampin

Capsules	150mg		ea
	300mg		ea

Rifampin and Isoniazid

Capsules	300mg/150mg		ea

Salmeterol Xinafoate

Inhalation aerosol	13Gm	Gm
Aerosol refill	13Gm	Gm

Restricted to claims submitted with dates of service from February 1, 1999 through July 31, 2005.

Inhalation powder	60s	ea

Salsalate

Tablets or capsules	500mg	ea
	750mg	ea

Restricted to use for arthritis.

Saquinavir

Capsules	200mg	ea
Tablets	500mg	ea

Restricted to use as combination therapy in the treatment of Human Immunodeficiency Virus (HIV) infection.

Tamoxifen Citrate

Tablets or capsules		ea

Tamsulosin HCL

Capsules	0.4mg	ea

Tazarotene

Topical cream or gel	0.05%	Gm
	0.1%	Gm

Restricted to use in the treatment of psoriasis.

Tegaserod

Tablets	2mg	ea
	6mg	ea

Restricted to use in women with irritable bowel syndrome.

Temazepam

Capsules	7.5mg	ea
	15mg	ea
	30mg	ea

Restricted to use in the treatment of insomnia.

Venlafaxine HCL

Capsules, extended release	37.5mg	ea
	75mg	ea
	150mg	ea

Verapamil HCL

Tablets	80mg	ea
	120mg	ea
Tablets, long acting	120mg	ea
	180mg	ea
	240mg	ea
Capsules, long acting	100mg	ea
	200mg	ea
	300mg	ea

Zidovudine

Tablets	300mg	ea
Capsules	100mg	ea
Liquid	50mg/5 cc	cc
Injection	10mg/cc	cc

Restricted to use as combination therapy in the treatment of Human Immunodeficiency Virus (HIV) infection.

Ziprasidone HCL

Capsules	20mg	ea
	40mg	ea
	60mg	ea
	80mg	ea

Restricted to individuals 6 years of age and older.

Zolpidem Tartrate

Tablets	5mg	ea
	10mg	ea
Tablets, extended release	6.25mg	ea
	12.5mg	ea

Restricted to use in the treatment of insomnia.

EXERCISE 2

Using the Bansal Formulary, what medications would you add to the formulary or discontinue if a pharmacy were located in the following geographic areas? Although formularies are not created on the basis of geographic areas, many pharmacies stock medications that are commonly used. In this case, the formulary will reflect the community that is using a particular pharmacy.

1. Retirement Facility:

_____

_____

_____

_____

2. HIV Clinic Pharmacy:

_____

_____

_____

_____

_____

3. Home Infusion Pharmacy:

_____

_____

_____

_____

_____

4. Pain Clinic Pharmacy:

_____

_____

_____

_____

_____

5. Psychiatric Facility:

_____

_____

_____

_____

_____

6. Alternative Medicine:

_____

_____

_____

_____

_____

Lab 21: Reading Medication Labels

OBJECTIVE

The student will learn to read and calculate drug labels for patient dosing.

INSTRUCTIONS

It is important to be able to read and understand prescription labels. In the following exercises, answer the questions in regards to the labels provided.

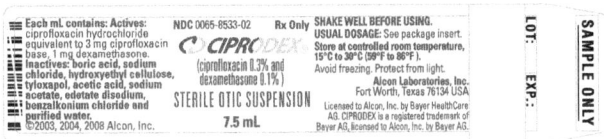

© Alcon Laboratories, Inc. Used with permission.

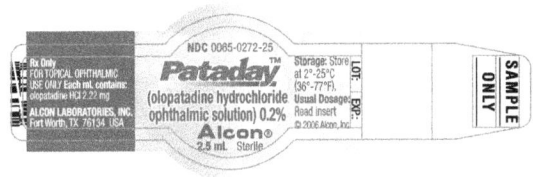

© Alcon Laboratories, Inc. Used with permission.

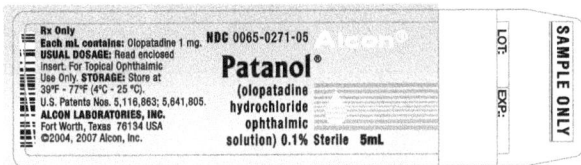

© Alcon Laboratories, Inc. Used with permission.

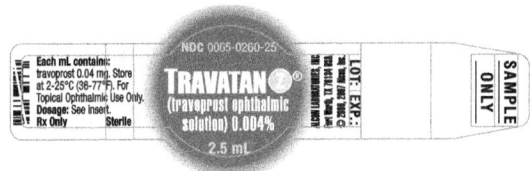

© Alcon Laboratories, Inc. Used with permission.

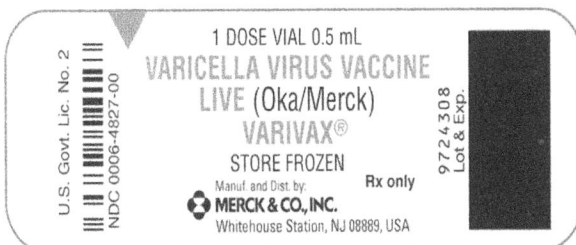

Courtesy of Merck & Co. Inc.

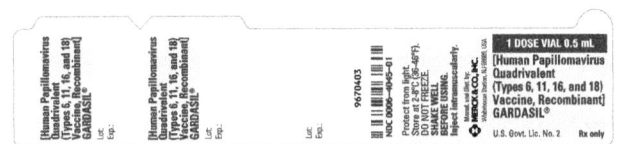

Courtesy of Merck & Co. Inc.

Hyzaar® 100-25
(Losartan Potassium-Hydrochlorothiazide Tablets)

Manufactured for:
MERCK & CO., INC., Whitehouse Station, NJ 08889, USA
By: MERCK SHARP & DOHME LTD.
Cramlington, Northumberland, UK NE23 3JU
Formulated in UK

Each tablet contains 100 mg losartan potassium and
25 mg hydrochlorothiazide.
Store at 25°C (77°F); excursions permitted to
15-30°C (59-86°F) [see USP Controlled Room
Temperature]. Keep container
tightly closed. Protect from
light.

NDC 0006-0747-54

USUAL ADULT DOSAGE: See accompanying circular.

Rx only

HYZAAR is a registered trademark of
E.I. du Pont de Nemours and Company,
Wilmington, DE

MRK 747

90 Tablets

Lot

9863000
90 | No. 3793

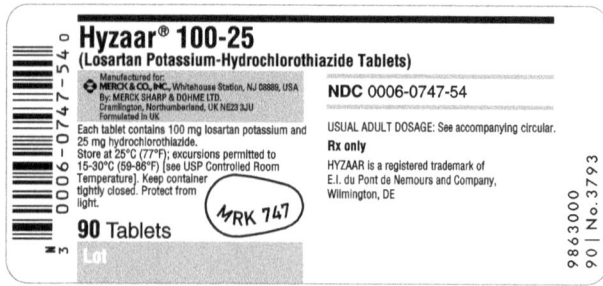

Courtesy of Merck & Co. Inc.

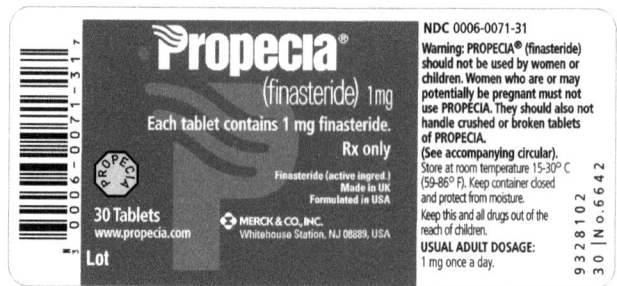

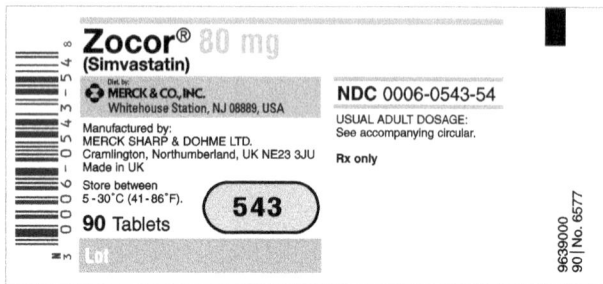

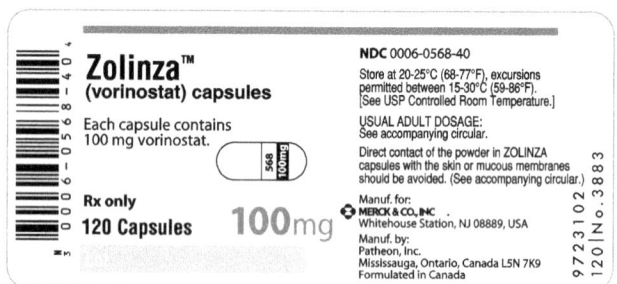

Propecia®
(finasteride) 1mg

Each tablet contains 1 mg finasteride.

Rx only

Finasteride (active ingred.)
Made in UK
Formulated in USA

30 Tablets
www.propecia.com

MERCK & CO., INC.
Whitehouse Station, NJ 08889, USA

Lot

NDC 0006-0071-31

Warning: PROPECIA® (finasteride)
should not be used by women or
children. Women who are or may
potentially be pregnant must not
use PROPECIA. They should also not
handle crushed or broken tablets
of PROPECIA.
(See accompanying circular).
Store at room temperature 15-30° C
(59-86° F). Keep container closed
and protect from moisture.
Keep this and all drugs out of the
reach of children.
USUAL ADULT DOSAGE:
1 mg once a day.

9328102
30 | No. 6642

Courtesy of Merck & Co. Inc.

Zocor® 80 mg
(Simvastatin)

Dist by:
MERCK & CO., INC.
Whitehouse Station, NJ 08889, USA

Manufactured by:
MERCK SHARP & DOHME LTD.
Cramlington, Northumberland, UK NE23 3JU
Made in UK

Store between
5-30°C (41-86°F).

90 Tablets

Lot

NDC 0006-0543-54

USUAL ADULT DOSAGE:
See accompanying circular.

Rx only

543

9639000
90 | No. 6577

Courtesy of Merck & Co. Inc.

Zolinza™
(vorinostat) capsules

Each capsule contains
100 mg vorinostat.

Rx only
120 Capsules   100mg

568
100mg

NDC 0006-0568-40

Store at 20-25°C (68-77°F), excursions
permitted between 15-30°C (59-86°F).
[See USP Controlled Room Temperature.]

USUAL ADULT DOSAGE:
See accompanying circular.

Direct contact of the powder in ZOLINZA
capsules with the skin or mucous membranes
should be avoided. (See accompanying circular.)

Manuf. for:
MERCK & CO., INC.
Whitehouse Station, NJ 08889, USA
Manuf. by:
Patheon, Inc.
Mississauga, Ontario, Canada L5N 7K9
Formulated in Canada

9723102
120 | No. 3883

Courtesy of Merck & Co. Inc.

1. Which medication has 0.1% Dexamethasone?

_____

2. There are _____ types of human papillomavirus quadrivalent. They are:

_____

3. Which medication(s) can be frozen?

_____

4. Which medication(s) is/are for topical ophthalmic use only?

_____

5. Which medication has the following NDC number: 0065-0260-25?

_____

6. Ciprodex comes in _____ ml.

7. There is an order for Zocor 40 mg bid × 30 days. Answer the following questions:

   a. How many tablets will the patient receive per dose? _____

   b. How many tablets will the patient receive for total therapy? _____

8. Which medication has the following written on their tablets: MRK747?

_____

9. What is the package size for Propecia?

_____

10. What is the generic for Zolinza?

_____

11. What is the strength of Losartan?

_____

12. How long can Pfizerpen be kept in the refrigerator before there is loss of potency?

_____

13. What is engraved on Zocar tablets?

_____

14. If 100,000 units/ml are needed, how many mls of diluents should be added?

_____

15. Who is the manufacturer for Ciprodex?

_____

16. After reconstitution, how long can Nebcin be stored?

_____

17. Pataday contains _____ mg of Olopatadine.

_____

18. What has been added during manufacturing in order to adjust the pH in Nebcin?

_____

19. Travatan contains _____ % (_____ gm) of medication.

_____

20. One dose of varicella virus vaccine equals _____ ml.

21. What is the NDC number for human papillomavirus quadrivalent?

_____

22. What is the average single IM injection for Pfizerpen one million units?

_____

23. How many medications has Merck produced?

_____

24. At what temperature should Zocor be stored?

_____

25. How many grams are in Nebcin?

_____

26. When adding 4 mls to penicillin G potassium, what will be the final units strength?

_____

27. At what temperature should Patanol be stored?

_____

28. What is the patent number for Patanol?

_____

29. Add _____ mls of _____ for a Nebcin injection.

30. What is the warning for taking Propecia?

_____

Lab 22: HIPAA

OBJECTIVE

The student will be able to understand HIPAA requirements for patient confidentiality.

What is HIPAA? HIPAA is the Health Insurance Portability & Accountability Act of 1996. HIPAA's goal is to improve efficiency/effectiveness of the healthcare system to protect privacy and security of individual health information.

In the pharmacy, all patient information must be kept strictly confidential. This includes:

- Patient profile info such as patient name, address, social security number, and other unique identifiers

- Patients' medical information such as diagnosis, allergies, medical history

- Prescriber information, DEA registration number, or license number

- Prescription info (i.e., drug names, strength, routine of administration, directions for use).

Employees in the pharmacy are not allowed to discuss the pharmacy information with anyone other than the patient, the prescriber or the other licensed practitioner caring for the patient, an authorized representative of the patient, a person who is authorized by law to receive information, or a pharmacist also serving the patient.

Patients are requested to sign an acknowledgment or receipt of notice of privacy practices, and they are given a copy of the privacy policy. Family members, i.e., spouse requesting patient information such as a profile or yearly reports for tax purposes must sign a disclosure authorization form that must also be signed by the patient. Many patients find this to be a hassle, but remember, it is the law. The penalty for wrongful disclosure of confidential information is 1 year imprisonment and/or a $50,000.00 fine!

Any materials containing confidential information (i.e., papers, labeled vials) must be disposed of properly in accordance with the law; most pharmacies have a shredding company dispose of confidential information marked for destruction. Receptacles are provided to store papers and vials, as you cannot just throw them in the garbage!

Go around to a few local pharmacies and ask for a HIPAA notice. Read it to become more familiar with your responsibility in keeping patient information confidential. Using HIPAA regulations, answer the following questions.

How would you handle the following scenarios?

1. A patient comes to the pharmacy counter and requests a copy of the prescriptions her husband had filled the previous year. She has her own driver's license for ID purposes. How do you respond?

_____

_____

_____

2. Mr. Jones has just left the pharmacy counter and you notice he left his credit card on the counter. You page "Mr. Jones, please return to the pharmacy." Is this a HIPAA violation?

_____

_____

_____

3. An employee is picking up their prescription for Viagra. You make a comment to another employee in confidence about this prescription. Is this a HIPAA violation?

_____

_____

_____

4. Mrs. Smith paid for her medication and doesn't want her prescription receipt. What do you do with it?

_____

_____

_____

5. Mr. Mad comes to the pharmacy counter and asks for his ex-wife's prescription record for the last 6 months. How do you respond?

_____

_____

_____

For more information about HIPAA go to www.hhs.gov/ocr/hipaa/.

Lab 23: Controlled Substance Log

OBJECTIVE

The student will learn how to complete a controlled substance log in order to record medications dispensed.

Controlled drugs, also referred to as scheduled drugs or narcotics, are prescription drugs placed in a scheduled class because of their potential for abuse and addictive properties. Prescriptions for scheduled drugs must be written on a special controlled substance form, faxed, or given orally except for schedule II narcotics. Define the following schedules of controlled medications.

EXERCISE 1

Using information from the DEA Web site, give examples of two medications in each of these drug classes. Give both brand and generic names. For a list of scheduled drugs you can visit the DEA Web site at www.dea.gov.

Schedule I

    1. Brand _____ Generic _____

    2. Brand _____ Generic _____

Schedule II

    1. Brand _____ Generic _____

    2. Brand _____ Generic _____

Schedule III

    1. Brand _____ Generic _____

    2. Brand _____ Generic _____

Schedule IV

    1. Brand _____ Generic _____

    2. Brand _____ Generic _____

Schedule V

1. Brand _____ Generic _____

2. Brand _____ Generic _____

EXERCISE 2

Using the prescriptions provided, complete the log sheet record for all the controlled medications dispensed in the pharmacy. For example, Jack Sparrow has a prescription for Methadone 10 mg, qty # 30. On hand the pharmacy has 150 tablets. If 30 are dispensed, then the remaining level is 120 tablets.

Table 23-1

Date	Name of Medication	Patient Name	# On Hand	# Dispensed	# Remaining
Example	Methadone 10 mg	Jack Sparrow	150	30	120
Example	Methadone 10 mg	John Doe	120	60	60
	Morphine 60 mg		333		
	Fentanyl		144		
	Oxycontin		268		
	Percodan		245		
	Ritalin 20 mg		422		
	Oxymorphone 5 mg		366		
	Morphine 90 mg		199		
	Dilaudid 8 mg		314		
	Methadone 5 mg		321		
	Fentanyl Patch 25 mcg		498		
	Percocet		288		

Date	Name of Medication	Patient Name	# On Hand	# Dispensed	# Remaining

Dr. Phull, H	Dr. Diver, Skye	Dr. Bansal, S	Dr. Perez, C
Dr. Mundian, K	Dr. Virdee, S	Dr. Climber, R	Dr. Racer, C
Dr. Dhillon, S	Dr. Chana, C	Dr. McDonald, R	Dr. Radia, K

Bansal Urgent Care

Name: _Jack Sparrow_ Date: _____

Address: _____

RX

Methadone 10mg   #30
   ⊤ qid prn pain

DAW ☐   Refill _NR_   MD _Perez, C._   Lic. No : _____
DEA# _____

Dr. Phull, H	Dr. Diver, Skye	Dr. Bansal, S	Dr. Perez, C
Dr. Mundian, K	Dr. Virdee, S	Dr. Climber, R	Dr. Racer, C
Dr. Dhillon, S	Dr. Chana, C	Dr. McDonald, R	Dr. Radia, K

Bansal Urgent Care

Name: _John Doe_ Date: _____

Address: _____

RX

Methadone 10mg #60
   TT qid prn pain
      NR   MD _____

DAW ☐   Refill _NR_   MD _____   Lic. No : _____
DEA# _____

Dr. Phull, H	Dr. Diver, Skye	Dr. Bansal, S	Dr. Perez, C
Dr. Mundian, K	Dr. Virdee, S	Dr. Climber, R	Dr. Racer, C
Dr. Dhillon, S	Dr. Chana, C	Dr. McDonald, R	Dr. Radia, K

Bansal Urgent Care

Name: _____ Date: _____

Address: _____

RX

Fentanyl Patch 25mcg   #7
apply 1 patch q 72 hrs for pain

DAW ☐   Refill _____   MD _Mundian, K._   Lic. No : _____
DEA# _____

Dr. Phull, H	Dr. Diver, Skye	Dr. Bansal, S	Dr. Perez, C
Dr. Mundian, K	Dr. Virdee, S	Dr. Climber, R	Dr. Racer, C
Dr. Dhillon, S	Dr. Chana, C	Dr. McDonald, R	Dr. Radia, K

Bansal Urgent Care

Name: _____ Date: _____

Address: _____

RX

Oxycontin 80mg #45
   ⊤ q 12 hrs post-op

DAW ☐   Refill _____   MD _____   Lic. No : _____
DEA# _____

Dr. Phull, H	Dr. Diver, Skye	Dr. Bansal, S	Dr. Perez, C
Dr. Mundian, K	Dr. Virdee, S	Dr. Climber, R	Dr. Racer, C
Dr. Dhillon, S	Dr. Chana, C	Dr. McDonald, R	Dr. Radia, K

Bansal Urgent Care

Name: _____ Date: _____
Address: _____
RX

Methadone 10 mg # 30
1 q 12 hrs for pain

DAW ☐   Refill _NR_   MD _(signature)_   Lic. No : _____
DEA# _____

Dr. Phull, H	Dr. Diver, Skye	Dr. Bansal, S	Dr. Perez, C
Dr. Mundian, K	Dr. Virdee, S	Dr. Climber, R	Dr. Racer, C
Dr. Dhillon, S	Dr. Chana, C	Dr. McDonald, R	Dr. Radia, K

Bansal Urgent Care

Name: _____ Date: _____
Address: _____
RX

Fentanyl Patch 25 mcg
apply 1 patch q 72 hrs

DAW ☐   Refill _____   MD _____   Lic. No : _____
DEA# _____

Dr. Phull, H	Dr. Diver, Skye	Dr. Bansal, S	Dr. Perez, C
Dr. Mundian, K	Dr. Virdee, S	Dr. Climber, R	Dr. Racer, C
Dr. Dhillon, S	Dr. Chana, C	Dr. McDonald, R	Dr. Radia, K

Bansal Urgent Care

Name: _____ Date: _____
Address: _____
RX

Methadone 5 mg # 30
1 tab q 8 hrs x 10d.

DAW ☐   Refill _NR_   MD _Chana C._   Lic. No : _____
DEA# _____

Dr. Phull, H	Dr. Diver, Skye	Dr. Bansal, S	Dr. Perez, C
Dr. Mundian, K	Dr. Virdee, S	Dr. Climber, R	Dr. Racer, C
Dr. Dhillon, S	Dr. Chana, C	Dr. McDonald, R	Dr. Radia, K

Bansal Urgent Care

Name: _____ Date: _____
Address: _____
RX

Morphine 90 mg caps # 60
II caps qd

DAW ☐   Refill _____   MD _Chana C._   Lic. No : _____
DEA# _____

Dr. Phull, H	Dr. Diver, Skye	Dr. Bansal, S	Dr. Perez, C
Dr. Mundian, K	Dr. Virdee, S	Dr. Climber, R	Dr. Racer, C
Dr. Dhillon, S	Dr. Chana, C	Dr. McDonald, R	Dr. Radia, K

Bansal Urgent Care

Name: _____ Date: _____
Address: _____
RX

Morphine 60mg caps # 30
T qd

DAW ☐   Refill _____   MD *Bansal*   Lic. No : _____
                          DEA# _____

Dr. Phull, H	Dr. Diver, Skye	Dr. Bansal, S	Dr. Perez, C
Dr. Mundian, K	Dr. Virdee, S	Dr. Climber, R	Dr. Racer, C
Dr. Dhillon, S	Dr. Chana, C	Dr. McDonald, R	Dr. Radia, K

Bansal Urgent Care

Name: _____ Date: _____
Address: _____
RX

Methadone 5mg #60
ii qd for severe pain

DAW ☐   Refill NR   MD *Bansal*   Lic. No : _____
                          DEA# _____

Dr. Phull, H	Dr. Diver, Skye	Dr. Bansal, S	Dr. Perez, C
Dr. Mundian, K	Dr. Virdee, S	Dr. Climber, R	Dr. Racer, C
Dr. Dhillon, S	Dr. Chana, C	Dr. McDonald, R	Dr. Radia, K

Bansal Urgent Care

Name: _____ Date: _____
Address: _____
RX

Morphine 60mg #120
TT caps bid ATC

DAW ☐   Refill _____   MD *Bansal*   Lic. No : _____
                          DEA# _____

Dr. Phull, H	Dr. Diver, Skye	Dr. Bansal, S	Dr. Perez, C
Dr. Mundian, K	Dr. Virdee, S	Dr. Climber, R	Dr. Racer, C
Dr. Dhillon, S	Dr. Chana, C	Dr. McDonald, R	Dr. Radia, K

Bansal Urgent Care

Name: _____ Date: _____
Address: _____
RX

Dilaudid 8mg #30
4mg q 4-6 hrs prn pain

DAW ☐   Refill _____   MD *Chana C.*   Lic. No : _____
                          DEA# _____

Dr. Phull, H	Dr. Diver, Skye	Dr. Bansal, S	Dr. Perez, C
Dr. Mundian, K	Dr. Virdee, S	Dr. Climber, R	Dr. Racer, C
Dr. Dhillon, S	Dr. Chana, C	Dr. McDonald, R	Dr. Radia, K

Bansal Urgent Care

Name: _____ Date: _____
Address: _____
RX

Percodan   # 30
   iq6hrs prn pain

DAW ☐   Refill _____   MD _____   Lic. No : _____
                           DEA# _____

Dr. Phull, H	Dr. Diver, Skye	Dr. Bansal, S	Dr. Perez, C
Dr. Mundian, K	Dr. Virdee, S	Dr. Climber, R	Dr. Racer, C
Dr. Dhillon, S	Dr. Chana, C	Dr. McDonald, R	Dr. Radia, K

Bansal Urgent Care

Name: _____ Date: _____
Address: _____
RX

Ritalin 20mg #100
   TT q8hrs

DAW ☐   Refill _____   MD H Phull   Lic. No : _____
                           DEA#

Dr. Phull, H	Dr. Diver, Skye	Dr. Bansal, S	Dr. Perez, C
Dr. Mundian, K	Dr. Virdee, S	Dr. Climber, R	Dr. Racer, C
Dr. Dhillon, S	Dr. Chana, C	Dr. McDonald, R	Dr. Radia, K

Bansal Urgent Care

Name: _____ Date: _____
Address: _____
RX

Dilaudid 8mg   #45
   4mg q4hrs prnp.

DAW ☐   Refill _____   MD _____   Lic. No : _____
                           DEA#

Dr. Phull, H	Dr. Diver, Skye	Dr. Bansal, S	Dr. Perez, C
Dr. Mundian, K	Dr. Virdee, S	Dr. Climber, R	Dr. Racer, C
Dr. Dhillon, S	Dr. Chana, C	Dr. McDonald, R	Dr. Radia, K

Bansal Urgent Care

Name: _____ Date: _____
Address: _____
RX

Ritalin 20mg # 60
   1 q 12hrs

DAW ☐   Refill _____   MD S Bansal   Lic. No : _____
                           DEA#

Dr. Phull, H	Dr. Diver, Skye	Dr. Bansal, S	Dr. Perez, C
Dr. Mundian, K	Dr. Virdee, S	Dr. Climber, R	Dr. Racer, C
Dr. Dhillon, S	Dr. Chana, C	Dr. McDonald, R	Dr. Radia, K

Bansal Urgent Care

Name: _____ Date: _____
Address: _____
RX

Percocet 2.5/325 #45
ī-īī tabs q6hrs NTE 12tabs

DAW ☐   Refill _____   MD *McDonald, R.*   Lic. No : _____
DEA# _____

FIGURE:

Dr. Phull, H	Dr. Diver, Skye	Dr. Bansal, S	Dr. Perez, C
Dr. Mundian, K	Dr. Virdee, S	Dr. Climber, R	Dr. Racer, C
Dr. Dhillon, S	Dr. Chana, C	Dr. McDonald, R	Dr. Radia, K

Bansal Urgent Care
1596 Antelope Canyons, Paige AZ 95874 (480) 458-8569 Fax: (480) 596-8248

Name: _____ Date: _____
Address: _____
RX

Percodan # 30
īqd prn pain

DAW ☐   Refill _____   MD *R Climber*   Lic. No : _____
DEA# _____

Dr. Phull, H	Dr. Diver, Skye	Dr. Bansal, S	Dr. Perez, C
Dr. Mundian, K	Dr. Virdee, S	Dr. Climber, R	Dr. Racer, C
Dr. Dhillon, S	Dr. Chana, C	Dr. McDonald, R	Dr. Radia, K

Bansal Urgent Care

Name: _____ Date: _____
Address: _____
RX

Percodan # 30
īqd prn pain

DAW ☐   Refill _____   MD *R Climber*   Lic. No : _____
DEA# _____

Dr. Phull, H	Dr. Diver, Skye	Dr. Bansal, S	Dr. Perez, C
Dr. Mundian, K	Dr. Virdee, S	Dr. Climber, R	Dr. Racer, C
Dr. Dhillon, S	Dr. Chana, C	Dr. McDonald, R	Dr. Radia, K

Bansal Urgent Care

Name: _____ Date: _____
Address: _____
RX

Oxycontin 80mg #30
one tab q24hrs prn P.

DAW ☐   Refill _____   MD *Virdee, S.*   Lic. No : _____
DEA# _____

Dr. Phull, H	Dr. Diver, Skye	Dr. Bansal, S	Dr. Perez, C
Dr. Mundian, K	Dr. Virdee, S	Dr. Climber, R	Dr. Racer, C
Dr. Dhillon, S	Dr. Chana, C	Dr. McDonald, R	Dr. Radia, K

Bansal Urgent Care

Name: _____ Date: _____
Address: _____
RX

Dilaudid 8mg   #40
8mg qid x10d

DAW ☐   Refill _____   MD _Racer, Car_   Lic. No : _____
DEA# _____

Dr. Phull, H	Dr. Diver, Skye	Dr. Bansal, S	Dr. Perez, C
Dr. Mundian, K	Dr. Virdee, S	Dr. Climber, R	Dr. Racer, C
Dr. Dhillon, S	Dr. Chana, C	Dr. McDonald, R	Dr. Radia, K

Bansal Urgent Care

Name: _____ Date: _____
Address: _____
RX

Ritalin 20mg # 30
T qd

DAW ☐   Refill _____   MD _Dhillon, S._   Lic. No : _____
DEA# _____

Dr. Phull, H	Dr. Diver, Skye	Dr. Bansal, S	Dr. Perez, C
Dr. Mundian, K	Dr. Virdee, S	Dr. Climber, R	Dr. Racer, C
Dr. Dhillon, S	Dr. Chana, C	Dr. McDonald, R	Dr. Radia, K

Bansal Urgent Care

Name: _____ Date: _____
Address: _____
RX

Oxymorphone 5mg #12
5mg pr q 4-6 hrs prn p

DAW ☐   Refill _____   MD _Radia, K._   Lic. No : _____
DEA# _____

Lab 24: Reading and Writing Prescriptions

OBJECTIVE

The student will learn how to recognize inaccuracies in a prescription and will also look at prescriptions from the point of view of a prescriber.

As a pharmacy technician in a retail setting, you are responsible for accepting written prescriptions and reviewing them for accurate information before entering the data into the computer. Written prescriptions must include the following:

- Patient's name

- Date

- Medication name and strength

- Quantity and directions

- Doctor's name and signature

Sometimes important information is not written on the prescription. In this case, the practitioner will be contacted by fax or phone to obtain the missing information. Also you will see DAW or DNS on some prescriptions. This means dispense as written or do not substitute. When this is noted on a prescription, the doctor is indicating that the drug prescribed should not be substituted with a generic drug.

INSTRUCTIONS

Look at the following prescriptions. Write in what is missing and circle any mistakes.

Dr. Phull, H	Dr. Diver, Skye	Dr. Bansal, S	Dr. Perez, C
Dr. Mundian, K	Dr. Virdee, S	Dr. Climber, R	Dr. Racer, C
Dr. Dhillon, S	Dr. Chana, C	Dr. McDonald, R	Dr. Radia, K

Bansal Urgent Care

Name: _Paper, antoilette_ Date: _2/23/08_
Address: _22 Skpoo Lane_
RX

SYNTHROID
#30
1 Qam

DAW ☐   Refill _3_   MD _____   Lic. No : _____
DEA#

Dr. Phull, H	Dr. Diver, Skye	Dr. Bansal, S	Dr. Perez, C
Dr. Mundian, K	Dr. Virdee, S	Dr. Climber, R	Dr. Racer, C
Dr. Dhillon, S	Dr. Chana, C	Dr. McDonald, R	Dr. Radia, K

Bansal Urgent Care

Name: _____ Date: _3/17/08_
Address: _____
RX

ATENLOL 50MG #30
1 TAB PO QD

DAW ☐   Refill _0_   MD _____   Lic. No : _____
DEA#

Dr. Phull, H	Dr. Diver, Skye	Dr. Bansal, S	Dr. Perez, C
Dr. Mundian, K	Dr. Virdee, S	Dr. Climber, R	Dr. Racer, C
Dr. Dhillon, S	Dr. Chana, C	Dr. McDonald, R	Dr. Radia, K

Bansal Urgent Care

Name: _A_ Date: _____
Address: _____
RX

Vicodin 500mg #145
III-II q____ X 4d

DAW ☐   Refill _6_   MD _Skinner_   Lic. No : _____
DEA#

Dr. Phull, H	Dr. Diver, Skye	Dr. Bansal, S	Dr. Perez, C
Dr. Mundian, K	Dr. Virdee, S	Dr. Climber, R	Dr. Racer, C
Dr. Dhillon, S	Dr. Chana, C	Dr. McDonald, R	Dr. Radia, K

Bansal Urgent Care

Name: _B_ Date: _____
Address: _____
RX

Benazepil 25mg XXX
Tbid

DAW ☐   Refill _13_   MD _McDonald_   Lic. No : _____
DEA#

```
Dr. Phull, H      Dr. Diver, Skye   Dr. Bansal, S      Dr. Perez, C
Dr. Mundian, K    Dr. Virdee, S     Dr. Climber, R     Dr. Racer, C
Dr. Dhillon, S    Dr. Chana, C      Dr. McDonald, R    Dr. Radia, K
```

Bansal Urgent Care

Name: _____C_____ Date: _____
Address: _____
RX

    Percoset 5mg # 300
        Tqd prn pain

DAW ☐   Refill _____ MD Climber, R   Lic. No :
                    DEA#

```
Dr. Phull, H      Dr. Diver, Skye   Dr. Bansal, S      Dr. Perez, C
Dr. Mundian, K    Dr. Virdee, S     Dr. Climber, R     Dr. Racer, C
Dr. Dhillon, S    Dr. Chana, C      Dr. McDonald, R    Dr. Radia, K
```

Bansal Urgent Care

Name: _____D_____ Date: _____
Address: _____
RX

    Coumadin 2mg # 30
        Tqd for BP

DAW ☐   Refill _2_ MD Radia, K.   Lic. No :
                    DEA#

```
Dr. Phull, H      Dr. Diver, Skye   Dr. Bansal, S      Dr. Perez, C
Dr. Mundian, K    Dr. Virdee, S     Dr. Climber, R     Dr. Racer, C
Dr. Dhillon, S    Dr. Chana, C      Dr. McDonald, R    Dr. Radia, K
```

Bansal Urgent Care

Name: _____E_____ Date: _____
Address: _____
RX

    Fentanyl Patches 10mcg # 7
    apply Tpatch q48hrs prn pain

DAW ☐   Refill _4_ MD Chana   Lic. No :
                    DEA#

```
Dr. Phull, H      Dr. Diver, Skye   Dr. Bansal, S      Dr. Perez, C
Dr. Mundian, K    Dr. Virdee, S     Dr. Climber, R     Dr. Racer, C
Dr. Dhillon, S    Dr. Chana, C      Dr. McDonald, R    Dr. Radia, K
```

Bansal Urgent Care

Name: _____F_____ Date: _____
Address: _____
RX

    Zoloft 150mg # 60
        T bid X 3months

DAW ☐   Refill _14_ MD Perez, C.   Lic. No :
                    DEA#

Occasionally you will come across a prescription that has been altered by the patient, most often the quantity or refills. The pharmacist should be notified immediately if you think a prescription has been tampered with. Look at the following prescriptions and determine which prescriptions are valid.

Dr. Phull, H	Dr. Diver, Skye	Dr. Bansal, S	Dr. Perez, C
Dr. Mundian, K	Dr. Virdee, S	Dr. Climber, R	Dr. Racer, C
Dr. Dhillon, S	Dr. Chana, C	Dr. McDonald, R	Dr. Radia, K

Bansal Urgent Care

Name: JONES, JIM   Date: 1/4/08
Address: PO BOX 99 OAKLAND CA
RX

NORCO 10/325 #150
1-2 Q4-6H
PRN PAIN

DAW ☐   Refill 10   MD _____   Lic. No: _____
DEA#

Valid   **Invalid**

Explain: _____

_____

Dr. Phull, H	Dr. Diver, Skye	Dr. Bansal, S	Dr. Perez, C
Dr. Mundian, K	Dr. Virdee, S	Dr. Climber, R	Dr. Racer, C
Dr. Dhillon, S	Dr. Chana, C	Dr. McDonald, R	Dr. Radia, K

Bansal Urgent Care

Name: BEAR, FUZZY   Date: 6/22/08
Address:
RX

Klonopin 1 mg
#30 1 TID

DAW ☐   Refill X   MD _____   Lic. No: _____
DEA#

Valid   **Invalid**

Explain: _____

_____

Dr. Phull, H	Dr. Diver, Skye	Dr. Bansal, S	Dr. Perez, C
Dr. Mundian, K	Dr. Virdee, S	Dr. Climber, R	Dr. Racer, C
Dr. Dhillon, S	Dr. Chana, C	Dr. McDonald, R	Dr. Radia, K

Bansal Urgent Care

Name: CANE, CANDY   Date: 2/2/08
Address: 31 NORTH POLE AVE
RX

SOMA 350MG #300
ī TID PRN

DAW ☐   Refill 6   MD _____   Lic. No: _____
DEA#

Valid   **Invalid**

Explain: _____

_____

```
Dr. Phull, H        Dr. Diver, Skye    Dr. Bansal, S      Dr. Perez, C
Dr. Mundian, K      Dr. Virdee, S      Dr. Climber, R     Dr. Racer, C
Dr. Dhillon, S      Dr. Chana, C       Dr. McDonald, R    Dr. Radia, K

Bansal Urgent Care

Name: Hannah Humina                     Date: 1/18/08
Address:
RX

                    #60   Tramadol 50mg
                          1 Twice Daily

DAW ☐      Refill  1      MD                    Lic. No :
                          DEA#
```

Valid   **Invalid**

Explain: _____

_____

Looking at the following prescriptions answer the following questions:

```
Dr. Phull, H        Dr. Diver, Skye    Dr. Bansal, S      Dr. Perez, C
Dr. Mundian, K      Dr. Virdee, S      Dr. Climber, R     Dr. Racer, C
Dr. Dhillon, S      Dr. Chana, C       Dr. McDonald, R    Dr. Radia, K

Bansal Urgent Care

Name: Annie Heinz                       Date: 6/7/08
Address: 71 St #21
RX

              Motrin 800mg  1 BID pc
              #60

DAW ☐      Refill  0      MD                    Lic. No :
                          DEA#
```

1. What is the drug that should be dispensed?

_____

_____

_____

2. Is a generic equivalent available?

_____

_____

_____

3. What are the directions to the patient in lay terms?

_____

_____

_____

Dr. Phull, H	Dr. Diver, Skye	Dr. Bansal, S	Dr. Perez, C
Dr. Mundian, K	Dr. Virdee, S	Dr. Climber, R	Dr. Racer, C
Dr. Dhillon, S	Dr. Chana, C	Dr. McDonald, R	Dr. Radia, K

Bansal Urgent Care

Name: _Paul, Pawley_____ Date: _5·10·07____
Address: _____
RX

GLUCOPHAGE 500mg
#60
BID

DAW ☐   Refill _1_   MD _____   Lic. No : ____
DEA#

1. What is the drug that should be dispensed?

_____

_____

_____

2. Is a generic equivalent available?

_____

_____

_____

3. What are the directions to the patient in lay terms?

_____

_____

_____

Play the role of the physician and write prescriptions for each of the patients below.

Patient 1

A 24-year-old male is diagnosed with genital herpes.

Dr. Phull, H	Dr. Diver, Skye	Dr. Bansal, S	Dr. Perez, C
Dr. Mundian, K	Dr. Virdee, S	Dr. Climber, R	Dr. Racer, C
Dr. Dhillon, S	Dr. Chana, C	Dr. McDonald, R	Dr. Radia, K

Bansal Urgent Care

Name: _____ Date: _____
Address: _____
RX

DAW ☐   Refill _____   MD _____ Lic. No : _____
                            DEA# _____

Patient 2

An 85-year-old female who has been diagnosed with angina pectoris.

Dr. Phull, H	Dr. Diver, Skye	Dr. Bansal, S	Dr. Perez, C
Dr. Mundian, K	Dr. Virdee, S	Dr. Climber, R	Dr. Racer, C
Dr. Dhillon, S	Dr. Chana, C	Dr. McDonald, R	Dr. Radia, K

Bansal Urgent Care

Name: _____ Date: _____
Address: _____
RX

DAW ☐   Refill _____   MD _____ Lic. No : _____
                            DEA# _____

Patient 3

This patient has elevated blood pressure due to water retention.

Dr. Phull, H	Dr. Diver, Skye	Dr. Bansal, S	Dr. Perez, C
Dr. Mundian, K	Dr. Virdee, S	Dr. Climber, R	Dr. Racer, C
Dr. Dhillon, S	Dr. Chana, C	Dr. McDonald, R	Dr. Radia, K

Bansal Urgent Care

Name: _____ Date: _____
Address: _____
RX

DAW ☐   Refill _____   MD _____ Lic. No : _____
                            DEA# _____

Patient 4

Female with type II diabetes and is insulin dependent.

```
Dr. Phull, H      Dr. Diver, Skye   Dr. Bansal, S     Dr. Perez, C
Dr. Mundian, K    Dr. Virdee, S     Dr. Climber, R    Dr. Racer, C
Dr. Dhillon, S    Dr. Chana, C      Dr. McDonald, R   Dr. Radia, K

Bansal Urgent Care

Name: _____   Date: _____
Address: _____
RX




DAW  ☐    Refill _____   MD _____   Lic. No : _____
                           DEA# _____
```

Patient 5

Male who is insulin dependent and has been diagnosed with erectile dysfunction.

```
Dr. Phull, H      Dr. Diver, Skye   Dr. Bansal, S     Dr. Perez, C
Dr. Mundian, K    Dr. Virdee, S     Dr. Climber, R    Dr. Racer, C
Dr. Dhillon, S    Dr. Chana, C      Dr. McDonald, R   Dr. Radia, K

Bansal Urgent Care

Name: _____   Date: _____
Address: _____
RX




DAW  ☐    Refill _____   MD _____   Lic. No : _____
                           DEA# _____
```

Patient 6

Female who has been diagnosed with estrogen deficiency. She suffers from irregular menstrual cycles.

```
Dr. Phull, H      Dr. Diver, Skye   Dr. Bansal, S     Dr. Perez, C
Dr. Mundian, K    Dr. Virdee, S     Dr. Climber, R    Dr. Racer, C
Dr. Dhillon, S    Dr. Chana, C      Dr. McDonald, R   Dr. Radia, K

Bansal Urgent Care

Name: _____   Date: _____
Address: _____
RX




DAW  ☐    Refill _____   MD _____   Lic. No : _____
                           DEA# _____
```

Patient 7

A 24-year-old female who has been diagnosed with Hepatitis C.

Dr. Phull, H	Dr. Diver, Skye	Dr. Bansal, S	Dr. Perez, C
Dr. Mundian, K	Dr. Virdee, S	Dr. Climber, R	Dr. Racer, C
Dr. Dhillon, S	Dr. Chana, C	Dr. McDonald, R	Dr. Radia, K

Bansal Urgent Care

Name: _____ Date: _____

Address: _____

RX

DAW ☐   Refill _____   MD _____   Lic. No : _____
                           DEA# _____

Patient 8

A 45-year-old male who has been diagnosed with TB. What is the medication regimen needed for this patient?

Dr. Phull, H	Dr. Diver, Skye	Dr. Bansal, S	Dr. Perez, C
Dr. Mundian, K	Dr. Virdee, S	Dr. Climber, R	Dr. Racer, C
Dr. Dhillon, S	Dr. Chana, C	Dr. McDonald, R	Dr. Radia, K

Bansal Urgent Care

Name: _____ Date: _____

Address: _____

RX

DAW ☐   Refill _____   MD _____   Lic. No : _____
                           DEA# _____

Patient 9

A 35-year-old female who has Candidiasis. This patient is currently on birth control.

Dr. Phull, H	Dr. Diver, Skye	Dr. Bansal, S	Dr. Perez, C
Dr. Mundian, K	Dr. Virdee, S	Dr. Climber, R	Dr. Racer, C
Dr. Dhillon, S	Dr. Chana, C	Dr. McDonald, R	Dr. Radia, K

Bansal Urgent Care

Name: _____ Date: _____

Address: _____

RX

DAW ☐   Refill _____   MD _____   Lic. No : _____
                           DEA# _____

Patient 10

A 50-year-old patient who has been diagnosed with HIV. The patient is also taking blood pressure medications, along with NTG when needed.

Dr. Phull, H	Dr. Diver, Skye	Dr. Bansal, S	Dr. Perez, C
Dr. Mundian, K	Dr. Virdee, S	Dr. Climber, R	Dr. Racer, C
Dr. Dhillon, S	Dr. Chana, C	Dr. McDonald, R	Dr. Radia, K

Bansal Urgent Care

Name: _____ Date: _____

Address: _____

RX

DAW ☐   Refill _____   MD _____   Lic. No : _____

DEA# _____

Name_____

Lab 25: Compounding

OBJECTIVE ──

Using base recipes, the student will learn how to compound different amounts.

PART 1 ──

The following are recipes that you will find in the Adventure Pharmacy. Calculate how many mls/grams the pharmacy technician will need in order to fill the written prescriptions. The recipes below are the original amounts; the student will need to alter the following amounts for each prescription. Please check with your instructor for expiration dates for each chemical.

Jasmine Diaper Rash Ointment

Vaseline	15g
Lavender Oil	5ml
Baby Oil	15ml
Cocoa Butter	2.5g
Total	37.5g

Simran Sunscreen

SPS 55	100mls
Lavender Oil	10mls
Aloe Vera	50mls
Xanthan Gum	150mls
Total	310mls

Navneil Body Cream

Water	10ml
Glycerin	100g
Cerna Lotion	150g
Citric Acid	15ml
Total	275g

Ria Baby Powder Lotion

Baby Oil	25mls
Baby Powder	5g
Sunscreen	25ml
Rose Oil	ii gtts
Total	55mls

Anisha Lotion

Cocoa Butter	5g
Aloe Vera	2.5g
Mineral Oil	15ml
Lavender	ii-iii gtts
Total	50g

Arvin Soothing Lotion

Dimethicone	15ml
Cetyl Alcohol	25ml
Shea Butter	1g
Glycerin	25ml
Total	66mls

Sabrina Body Spray

Alcohol	150mls
Water	75mls
Aloe Vera	150mls
Perfume	50mls
Total	425mls

Dr. Phull, H	Dr. Diver, Skye	Dr. Bansal, S	Dr. Perez, C
Dr. Mundian, K	Dr. Virdee, S	Dr. Climber, R	Dr. Racer, C
Dr. Dhillon, S	Dr. Chana, C	Dr. McDonald, R	Dr. Radia, K

Bansal Urgent Care

Name: _____ Date: _____
Address: _____
RX

Jasmine Diaper Rash Oint
AAA prn rash   #50g

DAW ☐   Refill ⑪   MD Phull, H   Lic. No. _____
DEA# _____

Table 25-1

Jasmine Diaper Rash							
Date	Ingredient	Amount Needed	Lot Number	Manufacturer	Expiration Date	Prepared By	Checked By
		Total					

Dr. Phull, H   Dr. Diver, Skye   Dr. Bansal, S   Dr. Perez, C
Dr. Mundian, K Dr. Virdee, S   Dr. Climber, R   Dr. Racer, C
Dr. Dhillon, S Dr. Chana, C   Dr. McDonald, R Dr. Radia, K

Bansal Urgent Care

Name: _____   Date: _____
Address: _____
RX

Ria Baby Powder lotion #100 mls
apply to hands as needed

DAW ☐   Refill ④   MD *Dhillon, S*   Lic. No : ____
                    DEA# _____

Table 25-2

				Ria Baby Powder Lotion			
Date	Ingredient	Amount Needed	Lot Number	Manufacturer	Expiration Date	Prepared By	Checked By
		Total					

Dr. Phull, H	Dr. Diver, Skye	Dr. Bansal, S	Dr. Perez, C
Dr. Mundian, K	Dr. Virdee, S	Dr. Climber, R	Dr. Racer, C
Dr. Dhillon, S	(Dr. Chana, C)	Dr. McDonald, R	Dr. Radia, K

Bansal Urgent Care

Name: _____   Date: _____

Address: _____

RX

Sabrina Body Spray # 125 mls

I—II sprays to body as needed

DAW ⊗   Refill (3)   MD *Chana, C*   Lic. No : _____
DEA# _____

Table 25-3

Sabrina Body Spray							
Date	Ingredient	Amount Needed	Lot Number	Manufacturer	Expiration Date	Prepared By	Checked By
		Total					

Dr. Phull, H	Dr. Diver, Skye	Dr. Bansal, S	Dr. Perez, C
Dr. Mundian, K	Dr. Virdee, S	Dr. Climber, R	Dr. Racer, C
Dr. Dhillon, S	Dr. Chana, C	Dr. McDonald, R	Dr. Radia, K

Bansal Urgent Care

Name: _____ Date: _____
Address: _____
RX

Simran Sunscreen #500 mls

apply to body prior to sun exposure

DAW ☐   Refill ④   MD *Virdee, S*   Lic. No : _____
DEA#

Table 25-4

Simran Sunscreen							
Date	Ingredient	Amount Needed	Lot Number	Manufacturer	Expiration Date	Prepared By	Checked By
		Total					

```
Dr. Phull, H      Dr. Diver, Skye   Dr. Bansal, S    Dr. Perez, C
Dr. Mundian, K    Dr. Virdee, S     Dr. Climber, R   Dr. Racer, C
Dr. Dhillon, S    Dr. Chana, C      Dr. McDonald, R  Dr. Radia, K

Bansal Urgent Care

Name: _____        Date: _____
Address: _____
RX
        Anisha Lotion #75g
        apply to dry skin qd

DAW  ∅    Refill (8)    MD Climber,R        Lic. No
                        DEA#
```

Table 25-5

Anisha Lotion							
Date	Ingredient	Amount Needed	Lot Number	Manufacturer	Expiration Date	Prepared By	Checked By
		Total					

Dr. Phull, H   Dr. Diver, Skye   Dr. Bansal, S   Dr. Perez, C
Dr. Mundian, K   Dr. Virdee, S   Dr. Climber, R   Dr. Racer, C
Dr. Dhillon, S   Dr. Chana, C   Dr. McDonald, R   Dr. Radia, K

Bansal Urgent Care

Name: _____   Date: _____
Address: _____
RX

Navneil Body Cream #300g
apply to feet as needed for dryness + cracked skin

DAW ☐   Refill ②   MD Racer, C   Lic. No :
DEA#

Table 25-6

Navneil Body Cream							
Date	Ingredient	Amount Needed	Lot Number	Manufacturer	Expiration Date	Prepared By	Checked By
		Total					

Dr. Phull, H   Dr. Diver, Skye   Dr. Bansal, S   Dr. Perez, C
Dr. Mundian, K   Dr. Virdee, S   Dr. Climber, R   Dr. Racer, C
Dr. Dhillon, S   Dr. Chana, C   Dr. McDonald, R   (Dr. Radia, K)

Bansal Urgent Care

Name: _____   Date: _____
Address: _____
RX

Arvin Soothing Lotion #
apply to sunburn after shower

DAW ☐   Refill (12)   MD Radia, K   Lic. No :
DEA#

Table 25-7

Arvin Soothing Lotion							
Date	Ingredient	Amount Needed	Lot Number	Manufacturer	Expiration Date	Prepared By	Checked By
		Total					

PART 2

Using the prescriptions provided, prepare the needed amount of capsules. Fill in the log chart of material used. For this exercise each capsule holds a maximum of 500mg. Inactive ingredient used is Sucrose.

Dr. Phull, H   Dr. Diver, Skye   Dr. Bansal, S   Dr. Perez, C
Dr. Mundian, K   Dr. Virdee, S   Dr. Climber, R   Dr. Racer, C
Dr. Dhillon, S   Dr. Chana, C   Dr. McDonald, R   Dr. Radia, K

Bansal Urgent Care

Name: Andrew Jackson   Date: 3/2/2008
Address: _____
RX

(Restoril 15mg) #45
(Tylenol 370mg) iqhs prn insomnia

DAW ☐   Refill Ø   MD Bansal   Lic. No :
DEA#

Dr. Phull, H	Dr. Diver, Skye	Dr. Bansal, S	Dr. Perez, C
Dr. Mundian, K	Dr. Virdee, S	Dr. Climber, R	Dr. Racer, C
Dr. Dhillon, S	Dr. Chana, C	Dr. McDonald, R	Dr. Radia, K

Bansal Urgent Care

Name: *Phillip Rayon*   Date: 5-6-03

Address: _____

RX

(Hydrocodone 10 mg
Motrin 200 mg) ī q 4 hrs prn pain #15

DAW ☐   Refill ∅   MD *Chana*   Lic. No :

DEA#

Dr. Phull, H	Dr. Diver, Skye	Dr. Bansal, S	Dr. Perez, C
Dr. Mundian, K	Dr. Virdee, S	Dr. Climber, R	Dr. Racer, C
Dr. Dhillon, S	Dr. Chana, C	Dr. McDonald, R	Dr. Radia, K

Bansal Urgent Care

Name: *Carol Jones*   Date: 3-3-03

Address: _____

RX

Atenolol 37mg #30 caps
ī qd x 30

DAW ☐   Refill ②   MD *Virdee*   Lic. No :

DEA#

Dr. Phull, H	Dr. Diver, Skye	Dr. Bansal, S	Dr. Perez, C
Dr. Mundian, K	Dr. Virdee, S	Dr. Climber, R	Dr. Racer, C
Dr. Dhillon, S	Dr. Chana, C	Dr. McDonald, R	Dr. Radia, K

Bansal Urgent Care

Name: *John Adams*   Date: 6-6-07

Address: _____

RX

Baclofen 15mg #60
ī bid x 30d

DAW ☐   Refill ③   MD *Diver, S.*   Lic. No :

DEA#

Dr. Phull, H	Dr. Diver, Skye	Dr. Bansal, S	Dr. Perez, C
Dr. Mundian, K	Dr. Virdee, S	Dr. Climber, R	Dr. Racer, C
Dr. Dhillon, S	Dr. Chana, C	Dr. McDonald, R	Dr. Radia, K

Bansal Urgent Care

Name: *Bubble Gum*   Date: 2-11-04

Address: _____

RX

Penicillin 300 mg #20 caps
ī bid x 10 d

DAW ☐   Refill ∅   MD *Dhillon*   Lic. No :

DEA#

Dr. Phull, H   Dr. Diver, Skye   Dr. Bansal, S   Dr. Perez, C
Dr. Mundian, K   Dr. Virdee, S   Dr. Climber, R   Dr. Racer, C
Dr. Dhillon, S   Dr. Chana, C   Dr. McDonald, R   Dr. Radia, K

Bansal Urgent Care

Name: _Baby Blue_   Date: _9-3-07_
Address: _____
RX

Compazine 175mg   # 30 Caps
T-ii q 4hrs prn N/V

DAW ☐   Refill _2_   MD _Bansal_   Lic. No : _____
                      DEA#

Patient Name	Capsules Needed	Ingredients Used	Amount Used

PART 3

Choose five chemicals and print a Material Safety Data Sheet from the manufacturer Spectrum. This can be obtained at www.spectrumchemical.com. Click on *fine chemicals in bulk*, then click on *Pharmaceutical Ingredients*. Pick the chemical you are researching and click on *MSDS*. Answer the following questions for each chemical.

1. What is the Toxicological Data on ingredients?

   a. _____

   b. _____

   c. _____

   d. _____

   e. _____

2. What are the potential acute health effects?

   a. _____

   b. _____

   c. _____

   d. _____

   e. _____

3. What should you do when there is eye and/or skin contact?

   a. _____

   b. _____

   c. _____

   d. _____

   e. _____

4. What should be done if the chemical in ingested?

   a. _____

   b. _____

   c. _____

   d. _____

   e. _____

5. What are the products of combustion?

a. _____

b. _____

c. _____

d. _____

e. _____

6. What are the fire fighting media?

a. _____

b. _____

c. _____

d. _____

e. _____

7. What precautions must be used when handling and storing?

a. _____

b. _____

c. _____

d. _____

e. _____

Name_____

Lab 26: Over-the-Counter Drugs

OBJECTIVE ——————————————————————————————————

To understand the average wholesale price mark-ups for pharmacy purchasing.

INSTRUCTIONS ——————————————————————————————

The U.S. Food and Drug Administration (FDA) determines whether medicines are prescription or nonprescription. The term prescription (Rx) refers to medicines that are safe and effective when used under a doctor's care. Nonprescription or OTC drugs are medicines FDA decides are safe and effective for use without a doctor's prescription. For this exercise, find one OTC medication that fits into each classification and fill in the required information. As a pharmacy owner you are to buy the medications from Jackies Distributing Co., in order to sell them in your pharmacy. You will have only $500,000 to spend and you must make a profit. Remember, some medications are fast movers and others are not, so buy accordingly.

Table 26-1

Classification	OTC Medication (Name and Active Ingredients)	AWP	Wholesale Acquisition Cost*	Total Amount Purchased/ Cost	Mark-Up	Processing Fee	Selling Price/ package	Profit/ per package
Acne			0.08% =					
Antipyretic			0.05% =					
Inflammation			0.02%					
Allergies			0.04%					
Antiemetics			0.01%					
Athlete's Foot			0.03%					
Antacids			0.04%					
Burns			0.05%					
Cold			0.02%					
Antidiarrhea			0.09%					
Heartburn			0.06%					
Eye Care			0.03%					
Ear Care			0.04%					
Gas, Flatulence, and Bloating			0.04%					
Hair Loss			0.10%					
Hemorrhoids			0.03%					
Insect Stings and Bites			0.06%					
Itching			0.09%					

Laxatives		0.08%				
Stool Softener		0.01%				
Cough Suppressant		0.10%				
Premenstrual Syndrome (PMS)		0.10%				
Pain Management		0.10%				
Poison Ivy/Oak		0.05%				
Antismoking		0.10%				
Sleep Aids and Stimulants		0.02%				
Sun Protection and Sunscreens		0.03%				
Warts		0.05%				
Weight Loss		0.07%				
Antifungal		0.09%				
Vitamins		0.11%				
Calcium Supplements		0.01%				
Topical Antibiotics		0.02%				
Total Amount Spent ($):					Projected Profit ($):	

*Wholesale Acquisition Cost—this is the manufacturer-suggested retail price. For each classification, you will receive a discount. For example, for acne medications a 0.08% discount was given off of the WAC.

Lab 27: Vitamins and Minerals

OBJECTIVE

To understand how minerals and vitamins work in the body as well as deficiency symptoms, overdose symptoms, and interactions.

INSTRUCTIONS

Complete the table with the following information:

- Vitamin—What is the vitamin prescribed for this deficiency?

- Generic—What is the generic name?

- Solubility—Is it fat or water soluble?

- RDA—What are the recommended daily allowances for men and women?

- Deficiency Symptoms—These are the symptoms one may have if they lack a vitamin.

- Physiological Indications (Method of Action)—How does this vitamin work in the body?

- Overdose Symptoms—What are the overdose symptoms for this vitamin?

- Interactions—Are there any interactions the patient should take into consideration?

Table 27-1

Vitamin	Generic	Solubility	RDA#	Deficiency Symptoms	Method of Action	Overdose Symptoms	Interactions
				Night blindness, dry cornea			
				Sensitivity to light, insomnia, ataxia, skin lesions, glossitis			
				Dark purplish dots on skin, tooth loss, pallor, sunken eyes			
				Unusual hemorrhage			
				Hemolytic anemia			

(continues)

Tingling, pricking, numbness of skin	Anemia	Weight loss, emotional disturbances, impaired sensory perception, weakness, pain in the limbs	Birth defects, neural tube defects	Alopecia, dermatitis, decreased appetite and growth, perosis, FLKS

Table 27-1 Continued

Vitamin	Generic	Solubility	RDA#	Deficiency Symptoms	Method of Action	Overdose Symptoms	Interactions
				Inhibition of DNA synthesis			
				Sore throat, throat mucosa, cheilosis, angular stomatitis, seborrheic dermatitis, decreased red blood count			
				Rickets and Osteomalacia			

*Men and women may differ in RDA requirements.

Lab 28: Basic Mathematical Conversions

OBJECTIVE

To complete mathematical conversions commonly used in the pharmacy.

Roman Numerals

I	=	1
V	=	5
X	=	10
L	=	50
C	=	100
D	=	500
M	=	1000

INSTRUCTIONS

Convert the following into Roman numerals.

1. 10   =

2. 24   =

3. 52   =

4. 485   =

5. 521   =

6. 732   =

7. 125   =

8. 526   =

9. 12   =

10. 15   =

11. 35   =

12. 75   =

13. 95   =

14. 11   =

15. 2   =

16. 85   =

17. 13   =

18. 58   =

19. 15   =

20. 54   =

Convert the following measurements.

1. 5mg   =   _____ mcg

2. 34mls   =   _____ oz

3. 652mls   =   _____ cups

4. 23g   =   _____ mgs

5. 749mls   =   _____ pts

6. 1.3gallons   =   _____ mls

7. 1L   =   _____ mls

8. 1g   =   _____ mcg

9. 1kg   =   _____ lbs

10. 357lbs   =   _____ g

11. 65T   =   _____ mls

12. 1tsp   =   _____ mls

13. 1pt   =   _____ mls

14. 1gr   =   _____ mg

15. 2.6pt   =   _____ qt

16. 6cups   =   _____ pts

17. 45fl. oz   =   _____ cups

18. 1dram   =   _____ mls

19. 1gtt   =   _____ mls

20. 5.6kg   =   _____ mg

21. 454lbs   =   _____ oz

22. 1,233,333mcg =   _____ kg

23. 1gal   =   _____ mls   =   _____ cups

24. 55,5638mls =   _____ gal   =   _____ cups

25. 67mls   =   _____ gtts

26. 786gr   =   _____ mg

27. 34kg   =   _____ lbs

28. 800lbs   =   _____ oz

29. 4KL   =   _____ mls

30. 34oz   =   _____ gr

31. 6drams   =   _____ tsp

32. 34qts   =   _____ mls

33. 45mls   =   _____ fl. oz

34. 137tsp   =   _____ cups

35. 35T   =   _____ mls

36. 1mg   =   _____ gms

37. 1000mg   =   _____ mcg

38. 1000mcg   =   _____ gr

39. 265gr   =   _____ oz

40. 45L   =   _____ KL

41. 45ml   =   _____ fl. oz

42. 2.5pt   =   _____ qt

43. 10 fl oz   =   _____ mls

44. 2.5kg   =   _____ lb

45. 8 L   =   _____ qt   =   _____ pt

46. 50 tbsp   =   _____ ml   =   _____ oz

47. 28g   =   _____ oz   =   _____ mg

48. 100gtts   =   _____ mls   =   _____ oz

49. 1floz   =   _____ T   =   _____ tsp

50. 2.2kg   =   _____ g   =   _____ lb

Lab 29: Dilutions and Stock Solutions

OBJECTIVE ————————————————————————————————

To be able to calculate dilutions and stock solutions.

INSTRUCTIONS ————————————————————————————————

Using the provided prescriptions, answer the following math questions in the space provided. Make any changes necessary to the quantity ordered in order to give the exact amount of medication to the patient. In some instances, the quantity may be left out and the student must calculate the amount needed. All stock solutions will be provided on the prescription.

1. Using the following prescriptions, find the percentage of active ingredient in the following preparations. Refer to prescription 1A for an example.

   1A Example:

Dr. Phull, H	Dr. Diver, Skye	Dr. Bansal, S	Dr. Perez, C
Dr. Mundian, K	Dr. Virdee, S	Dr. Climber, R	Dr. Racer, C
Dr. Dhillon, S	Dr. Chana, C	Dr. McDonald, R	Dr. Radia, K

Bansal Urgent Care

Name: _1A - EXAMPLE_   Date: _____

Address: _____

RX

0.5g of paxil in NS # ~~120mls~~ 50mls

1 tsp bid x5d $\frac{0.5g}{50mls} \times 100 = 1\%$

DAW ☐   Refill _4_   MD _____   Lic. No.: _____

DEA#

   1. Percentage strength is = 1%

   2. Qty changed to 50 because 1 tsp bid × 5 d = 5 × 2 × 5 = 50 mls

Dr. Phull, H　　Dr. Diver, Skye　Dr. Bansal, S　　Dr. Perez, C
Dr. Mundian, K　Dr. Virdee, S　　Dr. Climber, R　Dr. Racer, C
Dr. Dhillon, S　　Dr. Chana, C　　Dr. McDonald, R　Dr. Radia, K

Bansal Urgent Care

Name: _____1.0_____　　　Date: _____
Address: _____
RX

Motrin 1gm #30mls = %_____
π tsp prn HA

DAW ☐　　Refill ___2___　MD *Chana*　　Lic. No. : _____
　　　　　　　　　　　　　　DEA# _____

Dr. Phull, H　　Dr. Diver, Skye　Dr. Bansal, S　　Dr. Perez, C
Dr. Mundian, K　Dr. Virdee, S　　Dr. Climber, R　Dr. Racer, C
Dr. Dhillon, S　　Dr. Chana, C　　Dr. McDonald, R　Dr. Radia, K

Bansal Urgent Care

Name: _____1.1_____　　　Date: _____
Address: _____
RX

amoxil 0.25g in 250 mls = %_____
T tsp bid x10 d

DAW ☐　　Refill ___3___　MD *Climber, R*　　Lic. No. : _____
　　　　　　　　　　　　　　DEA#

Dr. Phull, H　　Dr. Diver, Skye　Dr. Bansal, S　　Dr. Perez, C
Dr. Mundian, K　Dr. Virdee, S　　Dr. Climber, R　Dr. Racer, C
Dr. Dhillon, S　　Dr. Chana, C　　Dr. McDonald, R　Dr. Radia, K

Bansal Urgent Care

Name: _____1.2_____　　　Date: _____
Address: _____
RX

TCN 0.8g #150mls = %_____
T tbsp bid x7d

DAW ☐　　Refill ___4___　MD *Racer, C*　　Lic. No. : _____
　　　　　　　　　　　　　　DEA# _____

Dr. Phuli, H   Dr. Diver, Skye   Dr. Bansal, S   Dr. Perez, C
Dr. Mundian, K Dr. Virdee, S   Dr. Climber, R   Dr. Racer, C
Dr. Dhillon, S   Dr. Chana, C   Dr. McDonald, R Dr. Radia, K

Bansal Urgent Care

Name: _1.3_ Date: _____
Address: _____
RX

    Cipro 3g   #250mls = % _____
    5mls qid x 14 d

DAW ☐   Refill _1_ MD _McDonald_ Lic. No: _____
    DEA# _____

Dr. Phuli, H   Dr. Diver, Skye   Dr. Bansal, S   Dr. Perez, C
Dr. Mundian, K Dr. Virdee, S   Dr. Climber, R   Dr. Racer, C
Dr. Dhillon, S   Dr. Chana, C   Dr. McDonald, R Dr. Radia, K

Bansal Urgent Care

Name: _1.4_ Date: _____
Address: _____
RX

    PCN 2.5g   #300mls = % _____
    i tsp q8hrs x10d

DAW ☐   Refill _2_ MD _Virdee, S._ Lic. No: _____
    DEA# _____

Dr. Phull, H   Dr. Diver, Skye   Dr. Bansal, S   Dr. Perez, C
Dr. Mundian, K Dr. Virdee, S   Dr. Climber, R   Dr. Racer, C
Dr. Dhillon, S   Dr. Chana, C   Dr. McDonald, R Dr. Radia, K

Bansal Urgent Care

Name: _1.5_   Date: _____
Address: _____
RX

Avelox 0.5g #25ml = % _____
Ttbsp bid x 4d

DAW ☐ Refill _4_ MD _Bansal_ Lic. No: _____
DEA#

Dr. Phull, H   Dr. Diver, Skye   Dr. Bansal, S   Dr. Perez, C
Dr. Mundian, K Dr. Virdee, S   Dr. Climber, R   Dr. Racer, C
Dr. Dhillon, S   Dr. Chana, C   Dr. McDonald, R Dr. Radia, K

Bansal Urgent Care

Name: _1.6_   Date: _____
Address: _____
RX

KiteK 0.3g #10ml = % _____
2ml qid x 2d

DAW ☒ Refill _4_ MD _Perez, Ch._ Lic. No: _____
DEA#

Dr. Phull, H   Dr. Diver, Skye   Dr. Bansal, S   Dr. Perez, C
Dr. Mundian, K Dr. Virdee, S   Dr. Climber, R   Dr. Racer, C
Dr. Dhillon, S   Dr. Chana, C   Dr. McDonald, R Dr. Radia, K

Bansal Urgent Care

Name: _1.7_   Date: _3/3/03_
Address: _____
RX

Amoxil 0.5g #150 mls % _____
5mls bid x 10d

DAW ☐ Refill _∅_ MD _SBansal_ Lic. No: _____
DEA#

Dr. Phull, H	Dr. Diver, Skye	Dr. Bansal, S	Dr. Perez, C
Dr. Mundian, K	Dr. Virdee, S	Dr. Climber, R	Dr. Racer, C
Dr. Dhillon, S	Dr. Chana, C	Dr. McDonald, R	Dr. Radia, K

Bansal Urgent Care

Name: _____ 1.8 _____ Date: _____

Address: _____

RX

Cefzil 0.4 g #

ī tsp q12hr X 30

% _____

DAW ☐   Refill 3   MD Diver, Skye   Lic. No : _____
DEA#

Dr. Phull, H	Dr. Diver, Skye	Dr. Bansal, S	Dr. Perez, C
Dr. Mundian, K	Dr. Virdee, S	Dr. Climber, R	Dr. Racer, C
Dr. Dhillon, S	Dr. Chana, C	Dr. McDonald, R	Dr. Radia, K

Bansal Urgent Care

Name: _____ 1.9 _____ Date: _____

Address: _____

RX

Biaxin 0.5 g #

īī tsp bid X 10d

= % _____

DAW ☐   Refill 3   MD Phull, H.   Lic. No : _____
DEA#

2. Using the following prescriptions, find the amount of grams or mg in each solution. Refer to prescription 11A for an example.

11A Example:

```
Dr. Phull, H        Dr. Diver, Skye   Dr. Bansal, S      Dr. Perez, C
Dr. Mundian, K      Dr. Virdee, S     Dr. Climber, R     Dr. Racer, C
Dr. Dhillon, S      Dr. Chana, C      Dr. McDonald, R    Dr. Radia, K

Bansal Urgent Care

Name:        11A – EXAMPLE              Date: _____
Address: _____
RX
       Minocin 9.5%    #250mls
                          ↪1100mls
       T tsp bid x 110 d          #g  104.5
                   9.5%
                   ────  x1100ml =
                   100%
DAW  ☐   Refill   0    MD  Dhillon, S          Lic. No :
                         DEA#
```

1. Amount of grams = 104.5 g

2. Qty changed to 1100 mls because 1 tsp bid × 110 d = 5 × 2 × 110 = 1100 mls

```
Dr. Phull, H        Dr. Diver, Skye   Dr. Bansal, S      Dr. Perez, C
Dr. Mundian, K      Dr. Virdee, S     Dr. Climber, R     Dr. Racer, C
Dr. Dhillon, S      Dr. Chana, C      Dr. McDonald, R    Dr. Radia, K

Bansal Urgent Care

Name:        12                        Date: _____
Address: _____
RX
       Omnicef 3.2%  # 500mls   #g_____
       15mls q4hrs x 12d

DAW  ☐   Refill   0    MD  Chana, C          Lic. No :
                         DEA#
```

```
┌─────────────────────────────────────────────────────────────┐
│ Dr. Phull, H     Dr. Diver, Skye   Dr. Bansal, S    Dr. Perez, C    │
│ Dr. Mundian, K   Dr. Virdee, S     Dr. Climber, R   Dr. Racer, C    │
│ Dr. Dhillon, S   Dr. Chana, C      Dr. McDonald, R  Dr. Radia, K    │
│                                                               │
│ Bansal Urgent Care                                            │
│                                                               │
│ Name: ____13_____    Date: _____        │
│ Address: _____         │
│ RX                                                            │
│        Acyclovir 1.5%  # 50mls  #g                            │
│     3mls qd X7d                                               │
│                                                               │
│                                                               │
│ DAW ☐      Refill __12__  MD  Radia, R.        Lic. No : ____ │
│                           DEA# _____                │
└─────────────────────────────────────────────────────────────┘
```

```
┌─────────────────────────────────────────────────────────────┐
│ Dr. Phull, H     Dr. Diver, Skye   Dr. Bansal, S    Dr. Perez, C    │
│ Dr. Mundian, K   Dr. Virdee, S     Dr. Climber, R   Dr. Racer, C    │
│ Dr. Dhillon, S   Dr. Chana, C      Dr. McDonald, R  Dr. Radia, K    │
│                                                               │
│ Bansal Urgent Care                                            │
│                                                               │
│ Name: ____14_____    Date: _____        │
│ Address: _____         │
│ RX                                                            │
│       Allopurinol 6%  #250mls                                 │
│     Ttsp bid X 30d.              #g                           │
│                                                               │
│                                                               │
│ DAW ☐      Refill __3__  MD Mundian, R.        Lic. No : ____ │
│                          DEA# _____                 │
└─────────────────────────────────────────────────────────────┘
```

Dr. Phull, H	Dr. Diver, Skye	Dr. Bansal, S	Dr. Perez, C
Dr. Mundian, K	Dr. Virdee, S	Dr. Climber, R	Dr. Racer, C
Dr. Dhillon, S	Dr. Chana, C	Dr. McDonald, R	Dr. Radia, K

Bansal Urgent Care

Name: _____15_____ Date: _____

Address: _____

RX

Topamax 7% #

TĪ tsp q12hrs X30d   mg_____

DAW ☐   Refill __4__ MD _Climber R._   Lic. No :_____

DEA#

Dr. Phull, H	Dr. Diver, Skye	Dr. Bansal, S	Dr. Perez, C
Dr. Mundian, K	Dr. Virdee, S	Dr. Climber, R	Dr. Racer, C
Dr. Dhillon, S	Dr. Chana, C	Dr. McDonald, R	Dr. Radia, K

Bansal Urgent Care

Name: _____16_____ Date: _____

Address: _____

RX

Xalantan 1% #5ml/s

TĪ gtts ou prn   g_____

DAW ☐   Refill __3__ MD _Phull, H._   Lic. No :_____

DEA#

Dr. Phull, H	Dr. Diver, Skye	Dr. Bansal, S	Dr. Perez, C
Dr. Mundian, K	Dr. Virdee, S	Dr. Climber, R	Dr. Racer, C
Dr. Dhillon, S	Dr. Chana, C	Dr. McDonald, R	Dr. Radia, K

Bansal Urgent Care

Name: _____17_____ Date: _____

Address: _____

RX

Levitra 8% # QS for 10 day

TĪ tbsp qd prn ed.   Supply

mg_____

DAW ☐   Refill __5__ MD _Dhillon, S._   Lic. No :_____

DEA#

Dr. Phull, H   Dr. Diver, Skye   Dr. Bansal, S   Dr. Perez, C
Dr. Mundian, K   Dr. Virdee, S   Dr. Climber, R   Dr. Racer, C
Dr. Dhillon, S   Dr. Chana, C   Dr. McDonald, R   Dr. Radia, K

Bansal Urgent Care

Name: ____18____   Date: _____
Address: _____
RX

Nexium 29% #

ɫɫɫɬsp q4hrs X 2d   mg_____

DAW ☐   Refill __5__   MD Dhillon, S.   Lic. No: ____
DEA# ____

Dr. Phull, H   Dr. Diver, Skye   Dr. Bansal, S   Dr. Perez, C
Dr. Mundian, K   Dr. Virdee, S   Dr. Climber, R   Dr. Racer, C
Dr. Dhillon, S   Dr. Chana, C   Dr. McDonald, R   Dr. Radia, K

Bansal Urgent Care

Name: ____19____   Date: _____
Address: _____
RX

Lamisil 13% # 200ml

apply 5mls qd X 40d   g_____

DAW ☐   Refill __6__   MD Bansal   Lic. No: ____
DEA# ____

```
Dr. Phull, H      Dr. Diver, Skye   Dr. Bansal, S      Dr. Perez, C
Dr. Mundian, K    Dr. Virdee, S     Dr. Climber, R     Dr. Racer, C
Dr. Dhillon, S    Dr. Chana, C      Dr. McDonald, R    Dr. Radia, K

Bansal Urgent Care

Name:_____20_____        Date:_____
Address:_____
RX
      abilify  5%   #
      T tsp  gram  x 30 d        mg_____


DAW  ☐     Refill_7____   MD  Bansal       Lic. No :_____
                         DEA#_____
```

3. Using the following prescriptions, calculate the amount of gms or mls that can be made from the stock on hand. Refer to 21A below for an example.

21A Example:

1. $0.5\% = 0.5\text{g} \times 1000 = 500 \text{ mg}$

2. $\dfrac{100\% \times 150 \text{ mg}}{500 \text{ mg}} = 30 \text{ g}$

```
Dr. Phull, H      Dr. Diver, Skye   Dr. Bansal, S      Dr. Perez, C
Dr. Mundian, K    Dr. Virdee, S     Dr. Climber, R     Dr. Racer, C
Dr. Dhillon, S    Dr. Chana, C      Dr. McDonald, R    Dr. Radia, K

Bansal Urgent Care

Name:_____21 A_____       Date:_____
Address:_____
RX
      Tac 0.5%   #  30 g
      apply prn to allergic reaction


DAW  ☐     Refill_4____   MD  Virdee      Lic. No :_____
                         DEA#_____
Stock 150 mg
```

```
Dr. Phull, H      Dr. Diver, Skye   Dr. Bansal, S     Dr. Perez, C
Dr. Mundian, K    Dr. Virdee, S     Dr. Climber, R    Dr. Racer, C
Dr. Dhillon, S    Dr. Chana, C      Dr. McDonald, R   Dr. Radia, K
```

Bansal Urgent Care

Name: _____22_____   Date: _____
Address: _____
RX

Benaclin 12% #_____
apply to face gom

DAW ☐   Refill 4   MD Radia R.   Lic. No: _____
                      DEA#
Stock 300mG

```
Dr. Phull, H      Dr. Diver, Skye   Dr. Bansal, S     Dr. Perez, C
Dr. Mundian, K    Dr. Virdee, S     Dr. Climber, R    Dr. Racer, C
Dr. Dhillon, S    Dr. Chana, C      Dr. McDonald, R   Dr. Radia, K
```

Bansal Urgent Care

Name: __23_____   Date: _____
Address: _____
RX

Nystatin 22% #_____
use as directed x 30 d

DAW ☐   Refill 2   MD McDonald, D.   Lic. No: _____
                      DEA#
Stock 155mG

Dr. Phull, H   Dr. Diver, Skye   Dr. Bansal, S   Dr. Perez, C
Dr. Mundian, K   Dr. Virdee, S   Dr. Climber, R   Dr. Racer, C
Dr. Dhillon, S   Dr. Chana, C   Dr. McDonald, R Dr. Radia, K

Bansal Urgent Care

Name: _____24_____ Date: _____
Address: _____
RX

Hydrocortisone 9% # _____
apply sparingly qd x 10d

DAW ☐   Refill 2   MD Racer, C.   Lic. No : _____
DEA# _____

Stock 0.5gm

Dr. Phull, H   Dr. Diver, Skye   Dr. Bansal, S   Dr. Perez, C
Dr. Mundian, K   Dr. Virdee, S   Dr. Climber, R   Dr. Racer, C
Dr. Dhillon, S   Dr. Chana, C   Dr. McDonald, R Dr. Radia, K

Bansal Urgent Care

Name: _____25_____ Date: _____
Address: _____
RX

acne cream 3% # _____
use daily

DAW ☐   Refill 2   MD Dhillon, S.   Lic. No : _____
DEA# _____

Stock 5 mg

Dr. Phull, H   Dr. Diver, Skye   Dr. Bansal, S   Dr. Perez, C
Dr. Mundian, K   Dr. Virdee, S   Dr. Climber, R   Dr. Racer, C
Dr. Dhillon, S   Dr. Chana, C   Dr. McDonald, R Dr. Radia, K

Bansal Urgent Care

Name: _____26_____ Date: _____
Address: _____
RX

Vaniqua 13% # _____
apply to skin (face) for wrinkles

DAW ☐   Refill 1   MD Perez, C.   Lic. No : _____
DEA# _____

Stock 10 mg

Dr. Phull, H   Dr. Diver, Skye   Dr. Bansal, S   Dr. Perez, C
Dr. Mundian, K   Dr. Virdee, S   Dr. Climber, R   Dr. Racer, C
Dr. Dhillon, S   Dr. Chana, C   Dr. McDonald, R   Dr. Radia, K

Bansal Urgent Care

Name: 27 ___ Date: ___
Address: ___
RX

Motrin 15% #_____ mLs
ī tsp bid prn pain

DAW ☐   Refill 2   MD Diver, Skye   Lic. No:
DEA#
Stock 30 mls

Dr. Phull, H   Dr. Diver, Skye   Dr. Bansal, S   Dr. Perez, C
Dr. Mundian, K   Dr. Virdee, S   Dr. Climber, R   Dr. Racer, C
Dr. Dhillon, S   Dr. Chana, C   Dr. McDonald, R   Dr. Radia, K

Bansal Urgent Care

Name: 28 ___ Date: ___
Address: ___
RX

Zyrtec 10% #_____ mLs
īī tsp qd

DAW ☐   Refill 2   MD Phull, H.   Lic. No:
DEA#
Stock 45 mls

Dr. Phull, H	Dr. Diver, Skye	Dr. Bansal, S	Dr. Perez, C
Dr. Mundian, K	Dr. Virdee, S	Dr. Climber, R	Dr. Racer, C
Dr. Dhillon, S	Dr. Chana, C	Dr. McDonald, R	Dr. Radia, K

Bansal Urgent Care

Name: 29   Date: _____
Address: _____
RX

Singulair 16% #_____ mLs
7.5 mls qd

DAW ☐   Refill ___1___   MD Mundian, K.   Lic. No: _____
                            DEA# _____

Stock 120 mls

Dr. Phull, H	Dr. Diver, Skye	Dr. Bansal, S	Dr. Perez, C
Dr. Mundian, K	Dr. Virdee, S	Dr. Climber, R	Dr. Racer, C
Dr. Dhillon, S	Dr. Chana, C	Dr. McDonald, R	Dr. Radia, K

Bansal Urgent Care

Name: 30   Date: _____
Address: _____
RX

allegra 7% #_____ mLs
T tsp bid

DAW ☐   Refill ___1___   MD Radia, R.   Lic. No: _____
                            DEA# _____

Stock 0.05 L

4. Using the following prescriptions, calculate the amount of mg and mls needed to fill the orders. Refer to prescription 51A for an example.

51A Example:

Dr. Phull, H	Dr. Diver, Skye	Dr. Bansal, S	Dr. Perez, C
Dr. Mundian, K	Dr. Virdee, S	Dr. Climber, R	Dr. Racer, C
Dr. Dhillon, S	Dr. Chana, C	Dr. McDonald, R	Dr. Radia, K

Bansal Urgent Care

Name: _____51A EXAMPLE_____ Date: _____
Address: _____
RX

Celebrex 1:300   Qty# _150 mls_
T tsp qd X30 d   mg _50_

DAW ☐   Refill _4_   MD _Mundian, K_   Lic. No : _____
         DEA#

1. Qty = 1 tsp qd × 30 = 5 mls × 1 × 30 days = 150 mls

2. $\dfrac{1}{300}$ = 0.003 × 150 mls = 0.1 g. Convert 0.1 g to mg = 0.1 × 1000 = 100 mg

Dr. Phull, H	Dr. Diver, Skye	Dr. Bansal, S	Dr. Perez, C
Dr. Mundian, K	Dr. Virdee, S	Dr. Climber, R	Dr. Racer, C
Dr. Dhillon, S	Dr. Chana, C	Dr. McDonald, R	Dr. Radia, K

Bansal Urgent Care

Name: _____52_____ Date: _____
Address: _____
RX

Relafin 2:3 Qty _____
8mls q4hrs x10 d   mg _____

DAW ☐   Refill _3_   MD _Dhillon, S._   Lic. No : _____
         DEA#

Dr. Phull, H	Dr. Diver, Skye	Dr. Bansal, S	Dr. Perez, C
Dr. Mundian, K	Dr. Virdee, S	Dr. Climber, R	Dr. Racer, C
Dr. Dhillon, S	Dr. Chana, C	Dr. McDonald, R	Dr. Radia, K

Bansal Urgent Care

Name: _____53_____ Date: _____

Address: _____

RX

Lunesta 1:400   Qty_____

T tsp qhs x 7d   mg_____

DAW ☐   Refill ___0___ MD _Perez, C_   Lic. No : _____
                        DEA# _____

Dr. Phull, H	Dr. Diver, Skye	Dr. Bansal, S	Dr. Perez, C
Dr. Mundian, K	Dr. Virdee, S	Dr. Climber, R	Dr. Racer, C
Dr. Dhillon, S	Dr. Chana, C	Dr. McDonald, R	Dr. Radia, K

Bansal Urgent Care

Name: _____54_____ Date: _____

Address: _____

RX

Atenolol 1:20   Qty_____

15mls qd x 80d

DAW ☐   Refill ___5___ MD _Perez, C_   Lic. No : _____
                        DEA# _____

Dr. Phull, H	Dr. Diver, Skye	Dr. Bansal, S	Dr. Perez, C
Dr. Mundian, K	Dr. Virdee, S	Dr. Climber, R	Dr. Racer, C
Dr. Dhillon, S	Dr. Chana, C	Dr. McDonald, R	Dr. Radia, K

Bansal Urgent Care

Name: _____55_____ Date: _____

Address: _____

RX

Zocor   1:500   Qty _300mls_

T tsp qid x 75d   mg_____

DAW ☐   Refill ___2___ MD _Bansal, S_   Lic. No : _____
                        DEA# _____

Dr. Phull, H	Dr. Diver, Skye	Dr. Bansal, S	Dr. Perez, C
Dr. Mundian, K	Dr. Virdee, S	Dr. Climber, R	Dr. Racer, C
Dr. Dhillon, S	Dr. Chana, C	Dr. McDonald, R	Dr. Radia, K

Bansal Urgent Care

Name: _____ 56 _____ Date: _____
Address: _____
RX

Viagra 11:4000   Qty_____
20mls qd   mg_____

DAW ☐   Refill 2 ___ MD _Mundian K._ Lic. No : ___
DEA# _____

Dr. Phull, H	Dr. Diver, Skye	Dr. Bansal, S	Dr. Perez, C
Dr. Mundian, K	Dr. Virdee, S	Dr. Climber, R	Dr. Racer, C
Dr. Dhillon, S	Dr. Chana, C	Dr. McDonald, R	Dr. Radia, K

Bansal Urgent Care

Name: _____ 57 _____ Date: _____
Address: _____
RX

Dilantin 1:10   Qty_____
7.5mls qid x 15d   mg_____

DAW ☐   Refill 3 ___ MD _Phull, H_ Lic. No : ___
DEA# _____

Dr. Phull, H	Dr. Diver, Skye	Dr. Bansal, S	Dr. Perez, C
Dr. Mundian, K	Dr. Virdee, S	Dr. Climber, R	Dr. Racer, C
Dr. Dhillon, S	Dr. Chana, C	Dr. McDonald, R	Dr. Radia, K

Bansal Urgent Care

Name: _____58_____ Date: _____

Address: _____

RX

Zoloft 4:1000   Qty _____

10mls qd X25d   mg _____

DAW ☐ Refill __1__ MD _Phull, H._ Lic. No: _____
DEA# _____

Dr. Phull, H	Dr. Diver, Skye	Dr. Bansal, S	Dr. Perez, C
Dr. Mundian, K	Dr. Virdee, S	Dr. Climber, R	Dr. Racer, C
Dr. Dhillon, S	Dr. Chana, C	Dr. McDonald, R	Dr. Radia, K

Bansal Urgent Care

Name: _____59_____ Date: _____

Address: _____

RX

Effexor 1:75   Qty _____

2 tbsp q 6hrs X10   mg _____

DAW ☐ Refill __1__ MD _Bansal S_ Lic. No: _____
DEA# _____

5. Using the following prescriptions, calculate the amount of mls needed to fill the orders.

   75A Example:

Dr. Phull, H	Dr. Diver, Skye	Dr. Bansal, S	Dr. Perez, C
Dr. Mundian, K	Dr. Virdee, S	Dr. Climber, R	Dr. Racer, C
Dr. Dhillon, S	Dr. Chana, C	Dr. McDonald, R	Dr. Radia, K

   Bansal Urgent Care

   Name: _75 A EXAMPLE_   Date: _____

   Address: _____

   RX

   Paxil 1:2000 Qty 40 oz
   IV tsp qid x 60d Stock 300 mls

   DAW ☑   Refill _2_   MD _Racer,C_   Lic. No: _____
   DEA#

   Stock 1:500 soln

   1. Qty needed = iv tsp qid × 60 days = 4 × 5 × 60 = 1200 mls or 40 fl. oz

   2. $\dfrac{1}{2000} = 0.0005$ and $\dfrac{1}{500} = 0.002$

   3. $\dfrac{0.005 \times 1200}{0.02} = 300\,mls$

   4. The technician needs 300 mls of the 1:500 stock solution to make 40 fl. oz of 1:2000 strength prescription.

Dr. Phull, H	Dr. Diver, Skye	Dr. Bansal, S	Dr. Perez, C
Dr. Mundian, K	Dr. Virdee, S	Dr. Climber, R	Dr. Racer, C
Dr. Dhillon, S	Dr. Chana, C	Dr. McDonald, R	Dr. Radia, K

   Bansal Urgent Care

   Name: _76_   Date: _____

   Address: _____

   RX

   _Amitriptiline 1:3000 Qty _____
   _9mls qid x 12d Stock mls _____

   DAW ☑   Refill _2_   MD _Bansal_   Lic. No: _____
   DEA#

   Stock 1:250 soln

Dr. Phull, H	Dr. Diver, Skye	Dr. Bansal, S	Dr. Perez, C
Dr. Mundian, K	Dr. Virdee, S	Dr. Climber, R	Dr. Racer, C
Dr. Dhillon, S	Dr. Chana, C	Dr. McDonald, R	Dr. Radia, K

Bansal Urgent Care

Name: 77   Date: _____
Address: _____
RX

Celexa 11:5000   Qty # 250 m/s
V mls q3hrs x12d   stock
needed   oz

DAW ☐   Refill 3   MD Chana, C   Lic. No:
DEA#
Stock 11:3000 soln

Dr. Phull, H	Dr. Diver, Skye	Dr. Bansal, S	Dr. Perez, C
Dr. Mundian, K	Dr. Virdee, S	Dr. Climber, R	Dr. Racer, C
Dr. Dhillon, S	Dr. Chana, C	Dr. McDonald, R	Dr. Radia, K

Bansal Urgent Care

Name: 78   Date: _____
Address: _____
RX

Lexapro 2:500   Qty _____
T tsp bid x 30d   Stock _____ oz

DAW ☒   Refill 7   MD McDonald, R   Lic. No:
DEA#
Stock 3:500

Dr. Phull, H	Dr. Diver, Skye	Dr. Bansal, S	Dr. Perez, C
Dr. Mundian, K	Dr. Virdee, S	Dr. Climber, R	Dr. Racer, C
Dr. Dhillon, S	Dr. Chana, C	Dr. McDonald, R	Dr. Radia, K

Bansal Urgent Care

Name: _____79_____   Date: _____
Address: _____
RX

PCN 1:250   Qty. 500 mls

III tsp bid X 15d   Stock needed _____ mL

DAW ☐   Refill _0_   MD _Dhillon, S._   Lic. No :
                        DEA#

Stock 2:500

Dr. Phull, H	Dr. Diver, Skye	Dr. Bansal, S	Dr. Perez, C
Dr. Mundian, K	Dr. Virdee, S	Dr. Climber, R	Dr. Racer, C
Dr. Dhillon, S	Dr. Chana, C	Dr. McDonald, R	Dr. Radia, K

Bansal Urgent Care

Name: _____80_____   Date: _____
Address: _____
RX

Soma 3:400   Qty 400 mls

T tbsp qd x45   stock needed _____07

DAW ☒   Refill _1_   MD _Climber, R._   Lic. No :
                        DEA#

Stock 4:1000

Dr. Phull, H	Dr. Diver, Skye	Dr. Bansal, S	Dr. Perez, C
Dr. Mundian, K	Dr. Virdee, S	Dr. Climber, R	Dr. Racer, C
Dr. Dhillon, S	Dr. Chana, C	Dr. McDonald, R	Dr. Radia, K

Bansal Urgent Care

Name: _____ 81 _____   Date: _____

Address: _____

RX

Plavix 0.5 : 100   Qty 100 mls

45 mls qam x 45d   Stock needed   oz

DAW ☐   Refill 3   MD Diver, Skye   Lic. No : _____

DEA# _____

Stock 0.2 : 3

Dr. Phull, H	Dr. Diver, Skye	Dr. Bansal, S	Dr. Perez, C
Dr. Mundian, K	Dr. Virdee, S	Dr. Climber, R	Dr. Racer, C
Dr. Dhillon, S	Dr. Chana, C	Dr. McDonald, R	Dr. Radia, K

Bansal Urgent Care

Name: _____ 82 _____   Date: _____

Address: _____

RX

Viagra 5 : 100   Qty

Ttsp qd prn x 5d   stick   oz

DAW ☐   Refill 5   MD McDonald, R.   Lic. No : _____

DEA# _____

stock 2 : 200

Dr. Phull, H	Dr. Diver, Skye	Dr. Bansal, S	Dr. Perez, C
Dr. Mundian, K	Dr. Virdee, S	Dr. Climber, R	Dr. Racer, C
Dr. Dhillon, S	Dr. Chana, C	Dr. McDonald, R	Dr. Radia, K

Bansal Urgent Care

Name: _83_ Date: _____
Address: _____

RX

Lescal   1:500   Qty

ттbsp qpm x 30d   Stock
                        needed _____ mL

DAW ☐   Refill __4__   MD _____   Lic. No : _____
                       DEA# _____

Dr. Phull, H	Dr. Diver, Skye	Dr. Bansal, S	Dr. Perez, C
Dr. Mundian, K	Dr. Virdee, S	Dr. Climber, R	Dr. Racer, C
Dr. Dhillon, S	Dr. Chana, C	Dr. McDonald, R	Dr. Radia, K

Bansal Urgent Care

Name: _84_ Date: _____
Address: _____

RX

Lamisil   1:400   Qty

apply 5mls to toes bid x 30d
                      stock needed _____ mL

DAW ☒   Refill __3__   MD _____   Lic. No : _____
                       DEA# _____

Lab 30: Reading Syringes

OBJECTIVE

By completing this exercise, the student will learn how to read different types of syringes.

INSTRUCTIONS

Draw a line on each syringe to the specified volume.

Part One: 10mls syringe

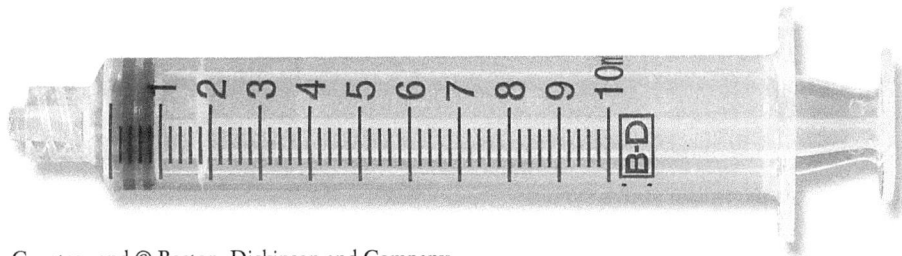

Courtesy and © Becton, Dickinson and Company

1. Draw a line to 3.8mls using the above syringe.

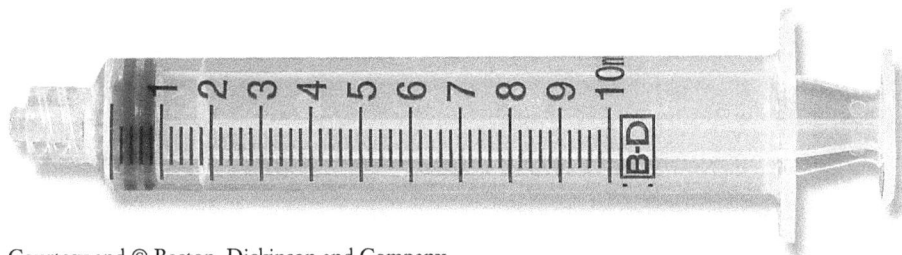

Courtesy and © Becton, Dickinson and Company

2. Draw a line to 6.4mls using the above syringe.

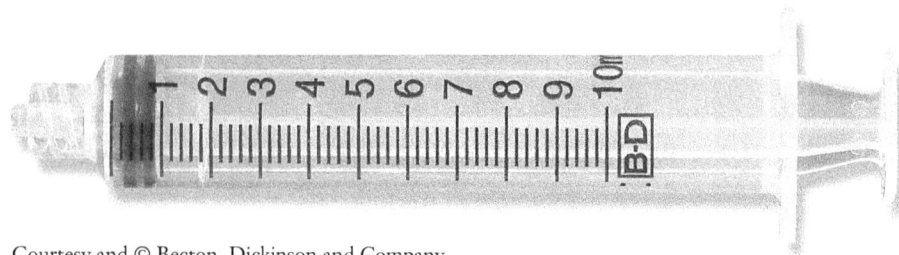

Courtesy and © Becton, Dickinson and Company

3. Draw a line 7.2mls using the above syringe.

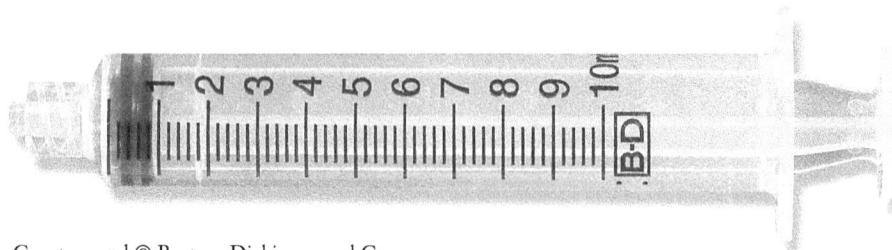

Courtesy and © Becton, Dickinson and Company

4. Draw a line to 2.2mls using the above syringe.

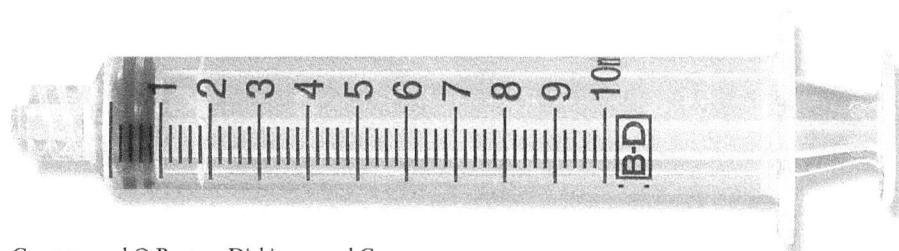

Courtesy and © Becton, Dickinson and Company

5. Draw a line to 5.6mls using the above syringe.

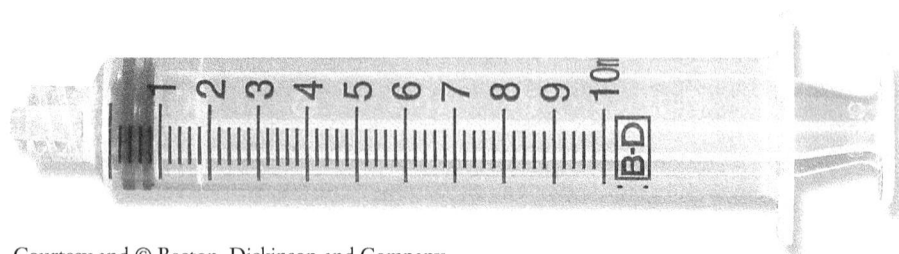

Courtesy and © Becton, Dickinson and Company

6. Draw a line to 9.6mls using the above syringe.

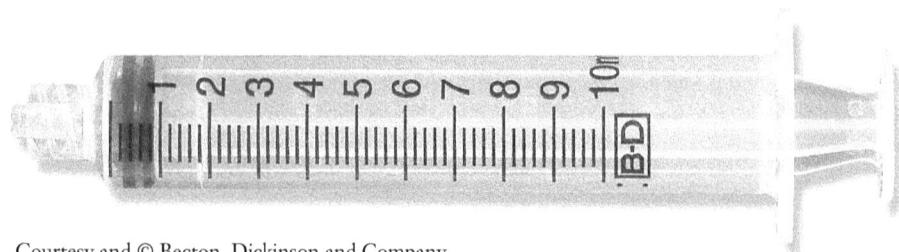

Courtesy and © Becton, Dickinson and Company

7. Draw a line to 3.8mls using the above syringe.

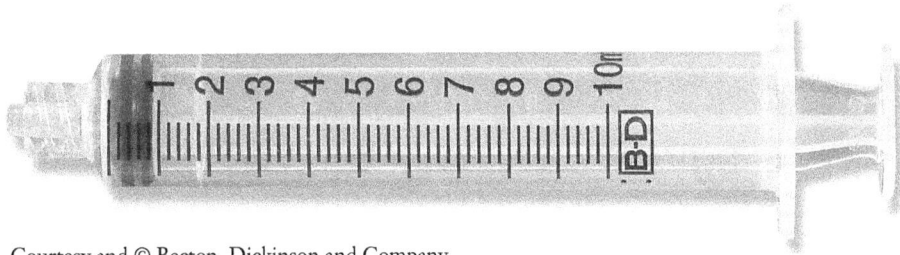

Courtesy and © Becton, Dickinson and Company

8. Draw a line to 10mls using the above syringe.

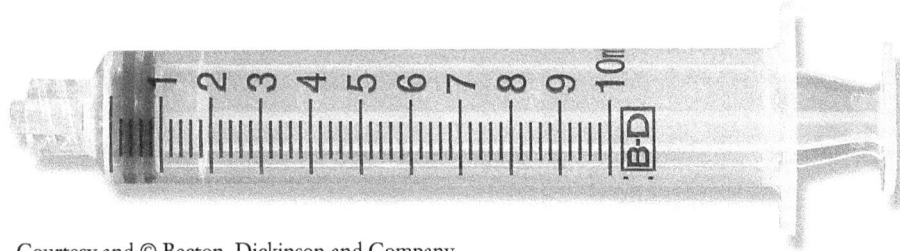

Courtesy and © Becton, Dickinson and Company

9. Draw a line to 3.8mls using the above syringe.

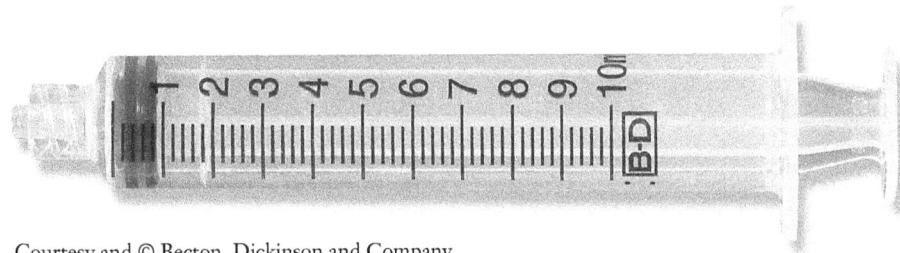

Courtesy and © Becton, Dickinson and Company

10. Draw a line to 1.4mls using the above syringe.

Part Two: 20mls syringe

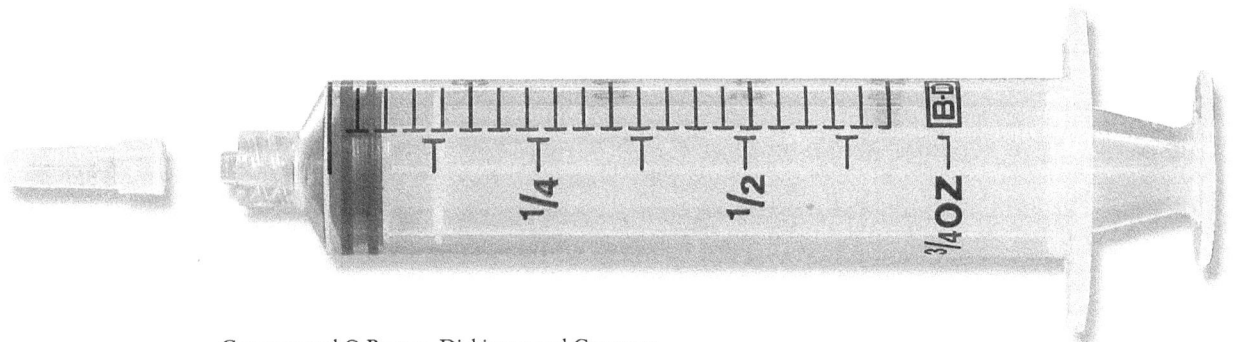

Courtesy and © Becton, Dickinson and Company

1. Draw a line to 12mls using the above syringe.

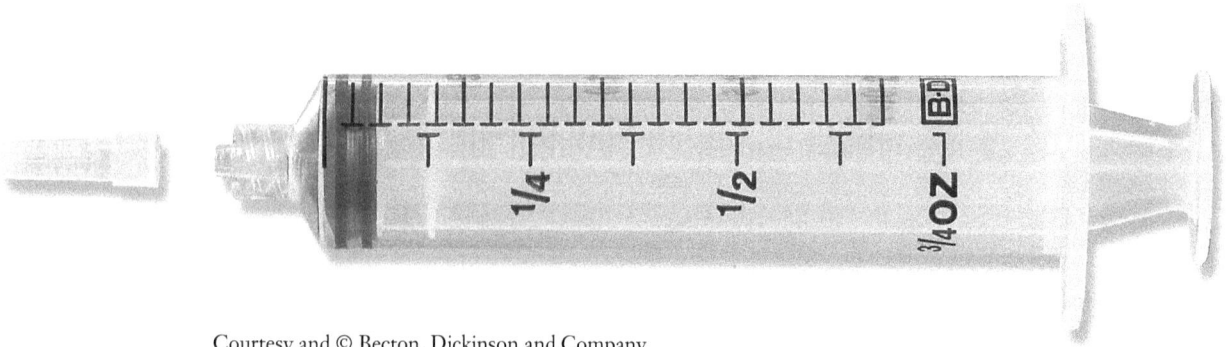

Courtesy and © Becton, Dickinson and Company

2. Draw a line to 7mls using the above syringe.

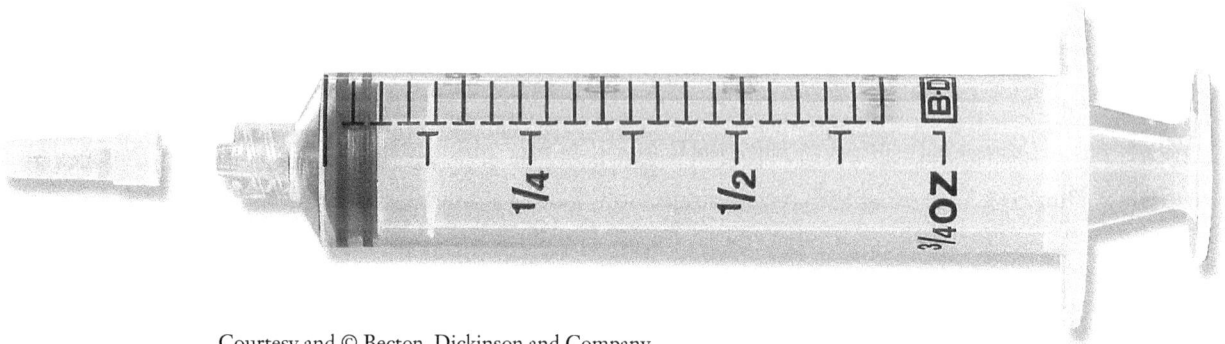

Courtesy and © Becton, Dickinson and Company

3. Draw a line to 9mls using the above syringe.

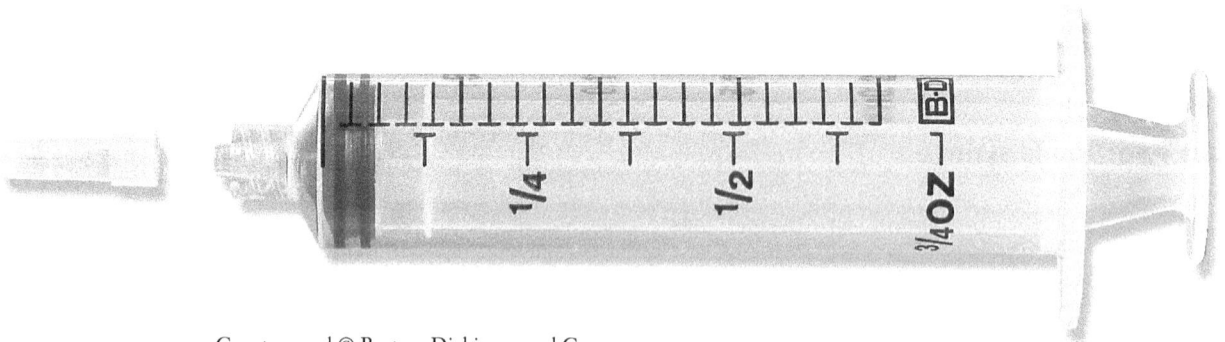

Courtesy and © Becton, Dickinson and Company

4. Draw a line to 17mls using the above syringe.

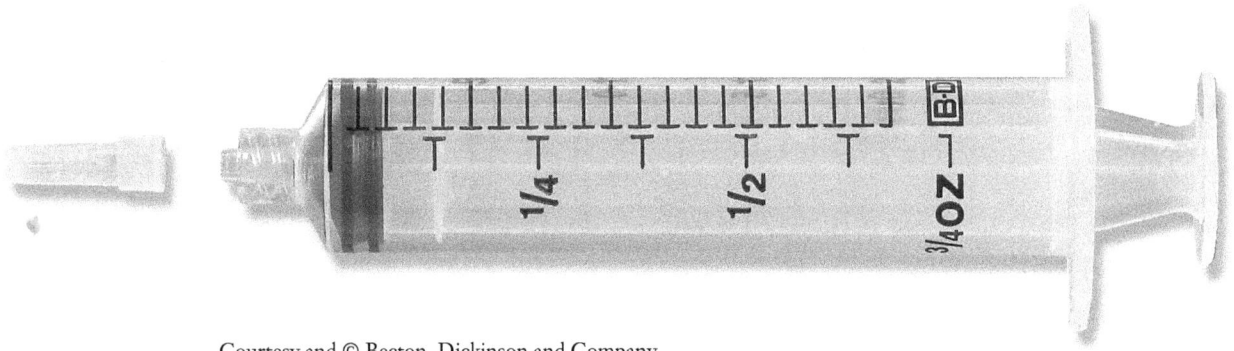

Courtesy and © Becton, Dickinson and Company

5. Draw a line to 13mls using the above syringe.

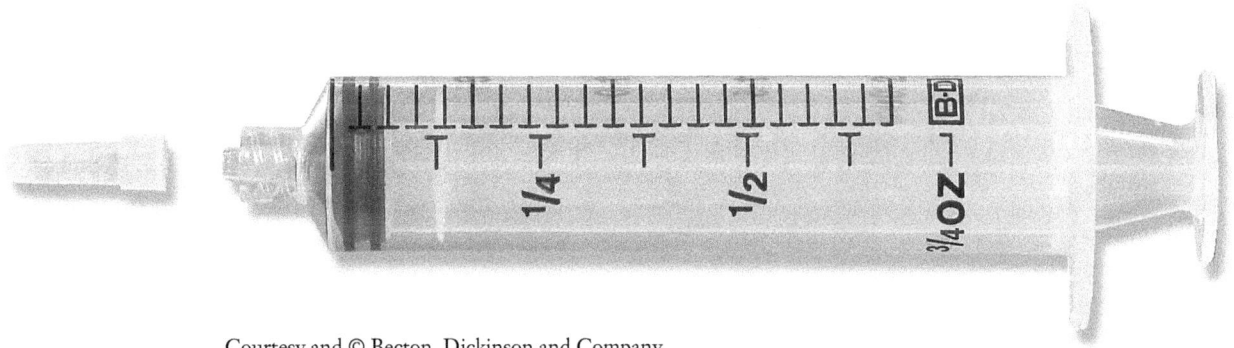

Courtesy and © Becton, Dickinson and Company

6. Draw a line to 4mls using the above syringe.

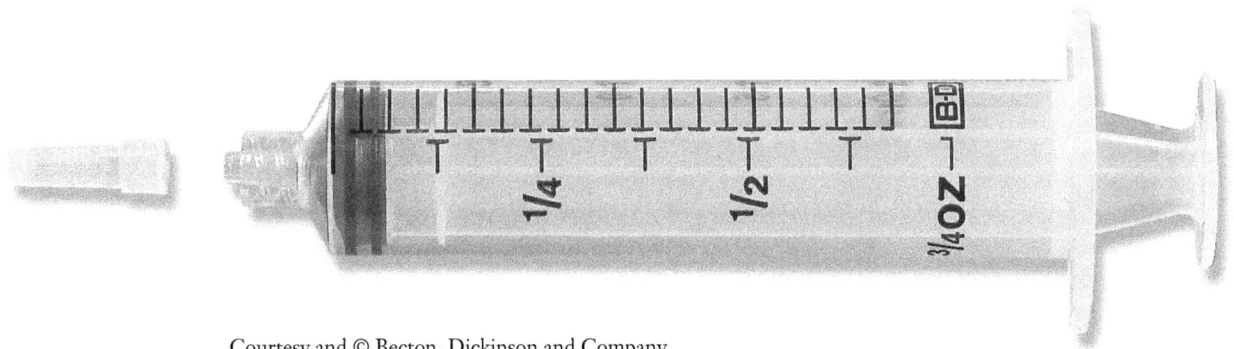

Courtesy and © Becton, Dickinson and Company

7. Draw a line to 2mls using the above syringe.

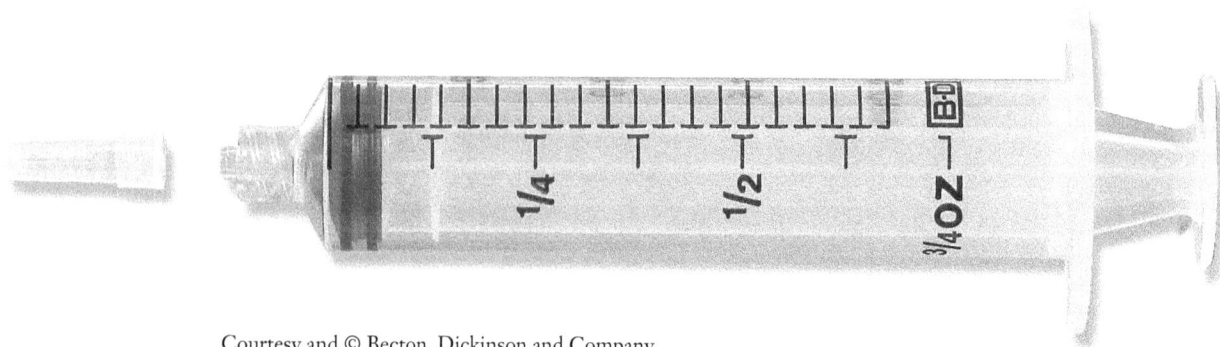

Courtesy and © Becton, Dickinson and Company

8. Draw a line to 20mls using the above syringe.

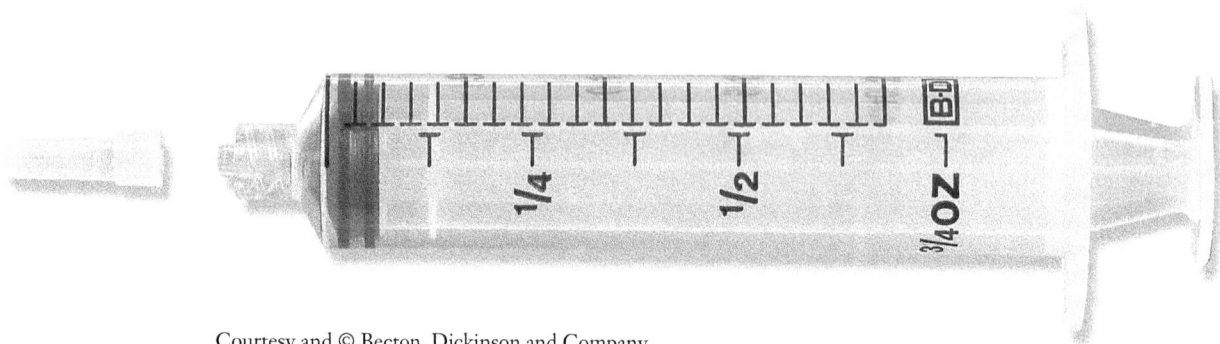

Courtesy and © Becton, Dickinson and Company

9. Draw a line to 10mls using the above syringe.

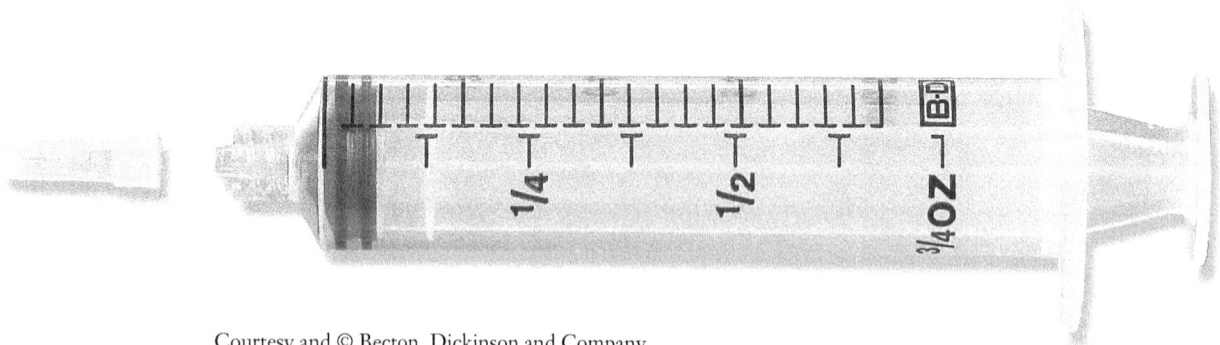

Courtesy and © Becton, Dickinson and Company

10. Draw a line to 15mls using the above syringe.

Part Three: 30mls syringe

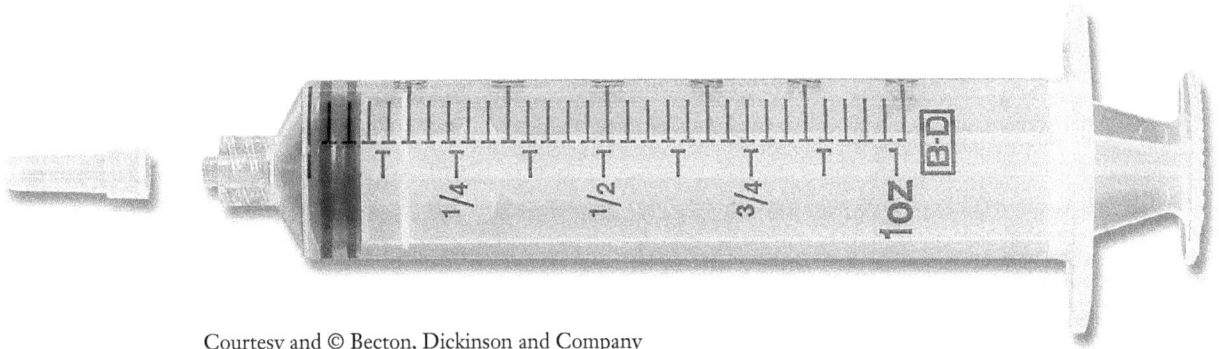

Courtesy and © Becton, Dickinson and Company

1. Draw a line to 25mls using the above syringe.

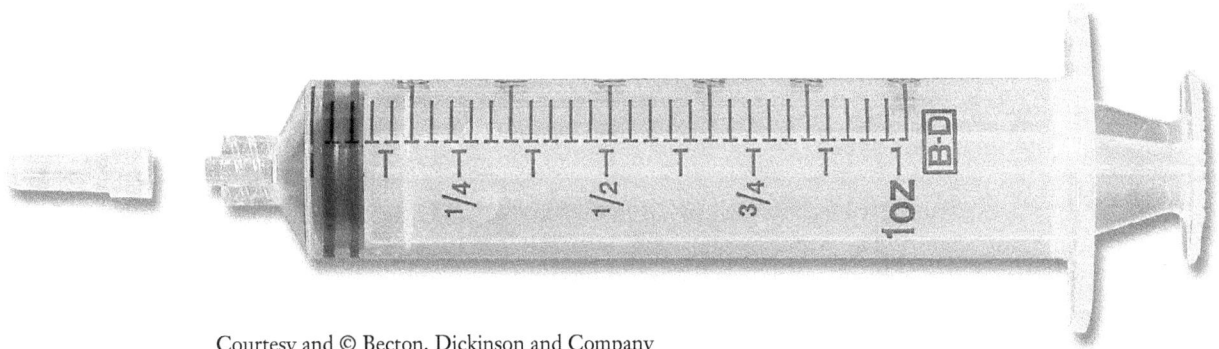

Courtesy and © Becton, Dickinson and Company

2. Draw a line to 15mls using the above syringe.

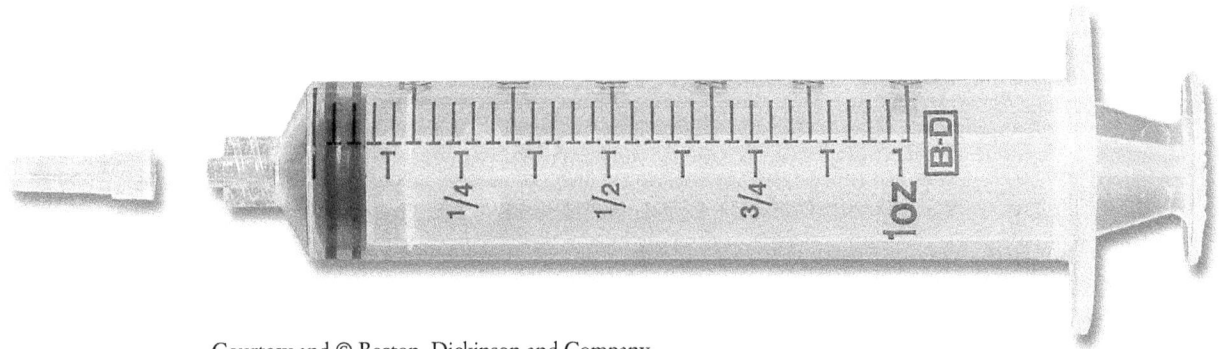

Courtesy and © Becton, Dickinson and Company

3. Draw a line to 10mls using the above syringe.

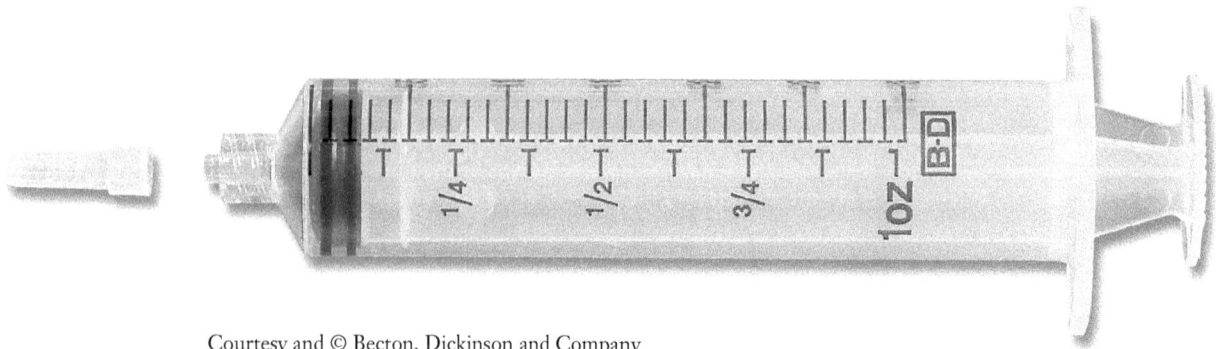

Courtesy and © Becton, Dickinson and Company

4. Draw a line to 30mls using the above syringe.

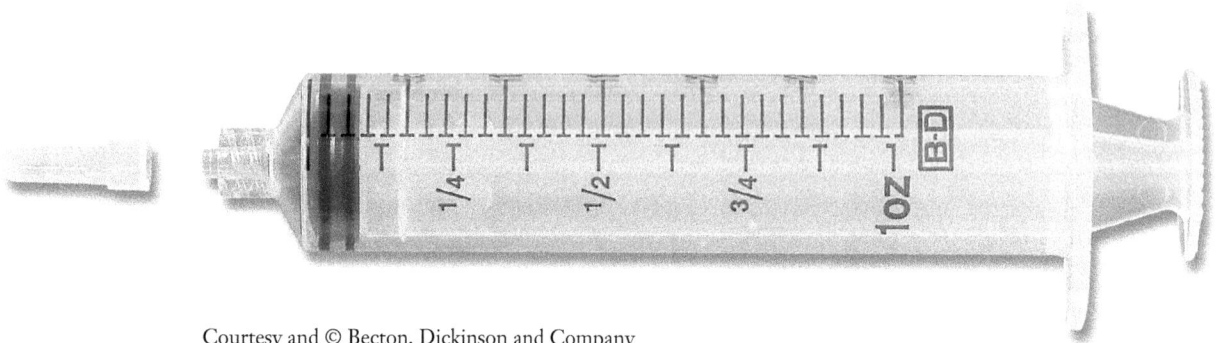

Courtesy and © Becton, Dickinson and Company

5. Draw a line to 24mls using the above syringe.

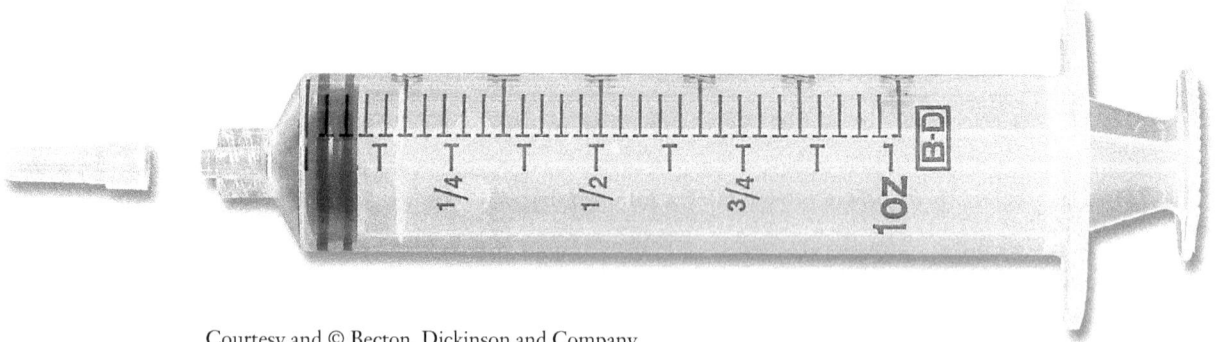

Courtesy and © Becton, Dickinson and Company

6. Draw a line to 5mls using the above syringe.

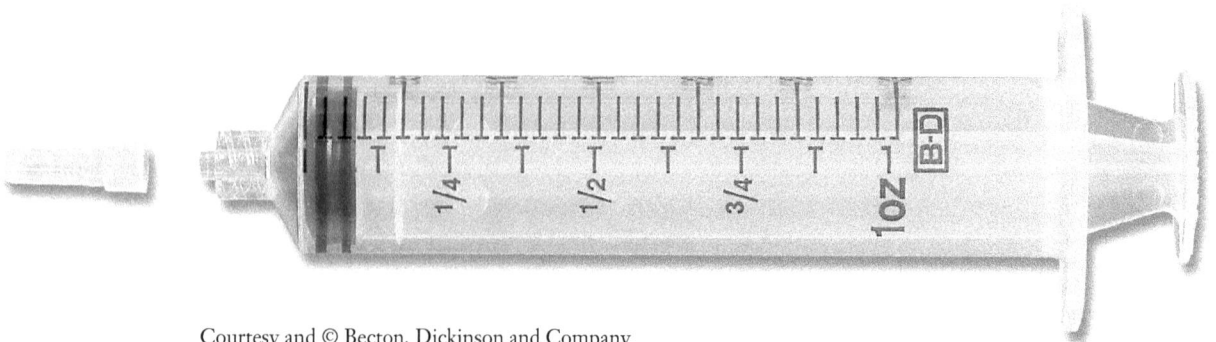

Courtesy and © Becton, Dickinson and Company

7. Draw a line to 0.6mls using the above syringe.

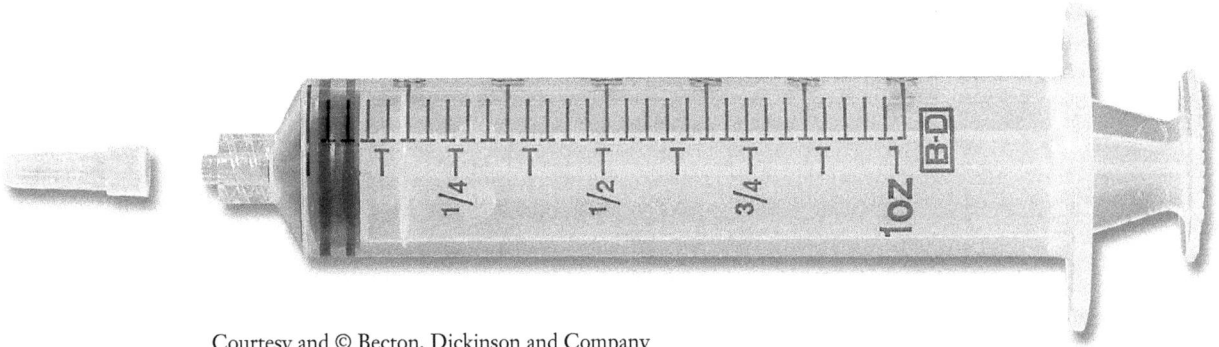

Courtesy and © Becton, Dickinson and Company

8. Draw a line to 18mls using the above syringe.

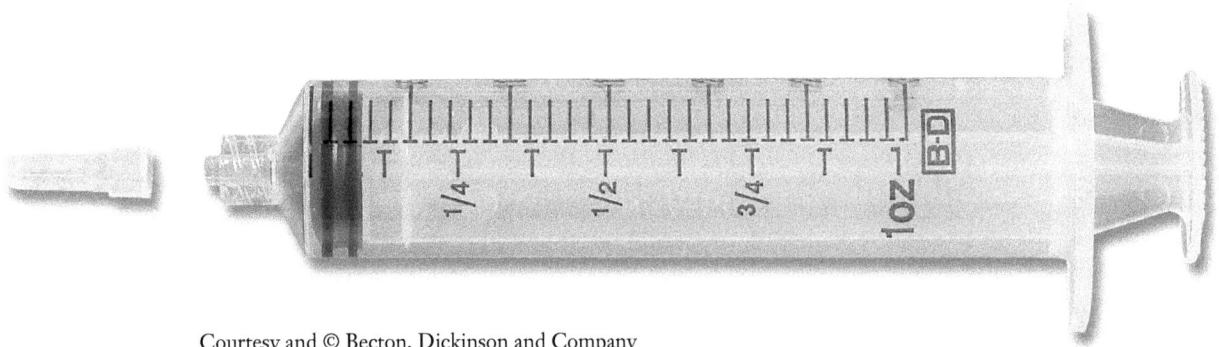

Courtesy and © Becton, Dickinson and Company

9. Draw a line to 5.8mls using the above syringe.

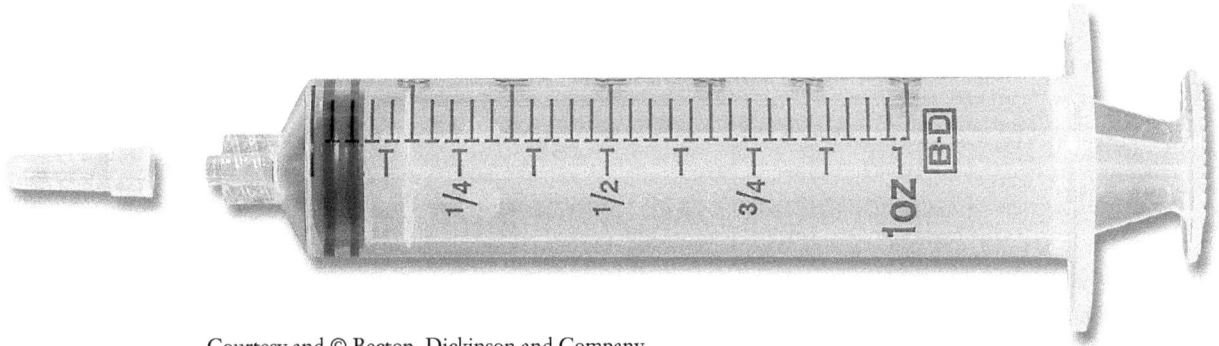

Courtesy and © Becton, Dickinson and Company

10. Draw a line to 12.4mls using the above syringe.

Part Four: 60mls syringe

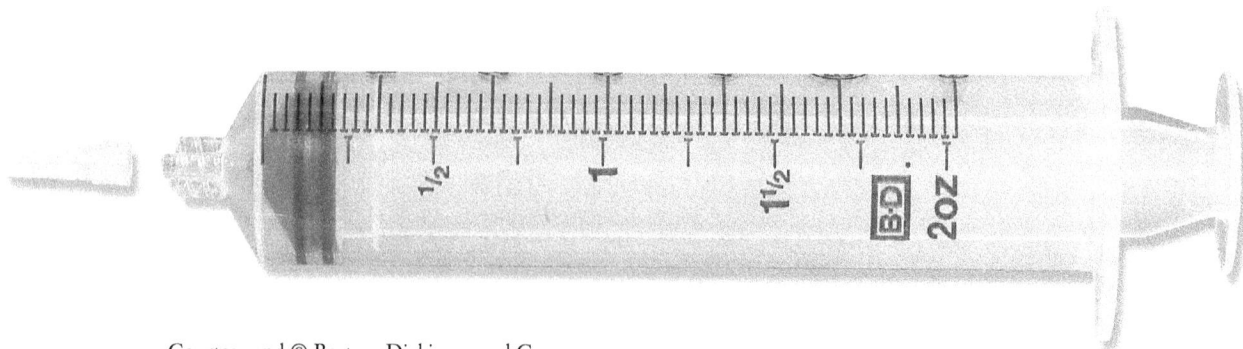

Courtesy and © Becton, Dickinson and Company

1. Draw a line to 20mls using the above syringe.

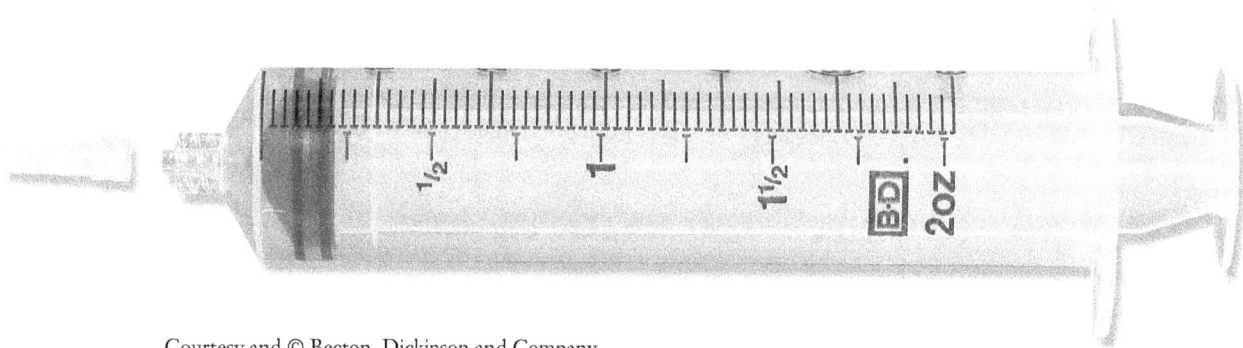

Courtesy and © Becton, Dickinson and Company

2. Draw a line to 35mls using the above syringe.

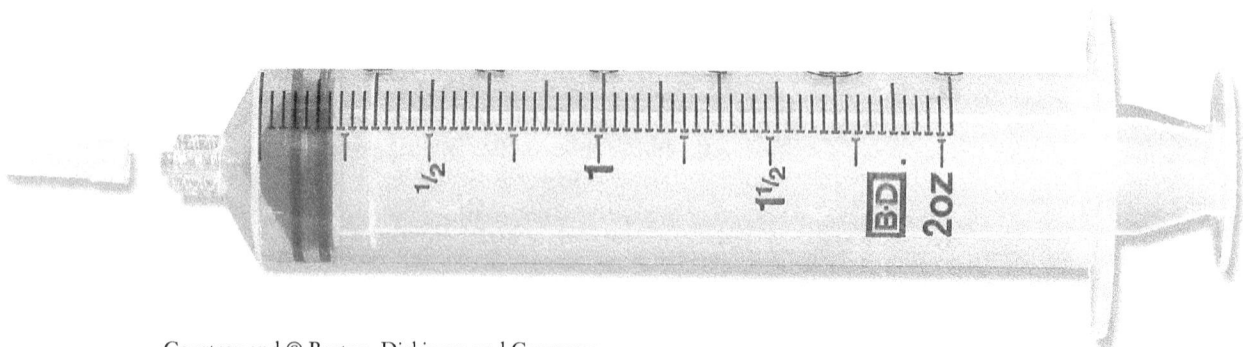

Courtesy and © Becton, Dickinson and Company

3. Draw a line to 22mls using the above syringe.

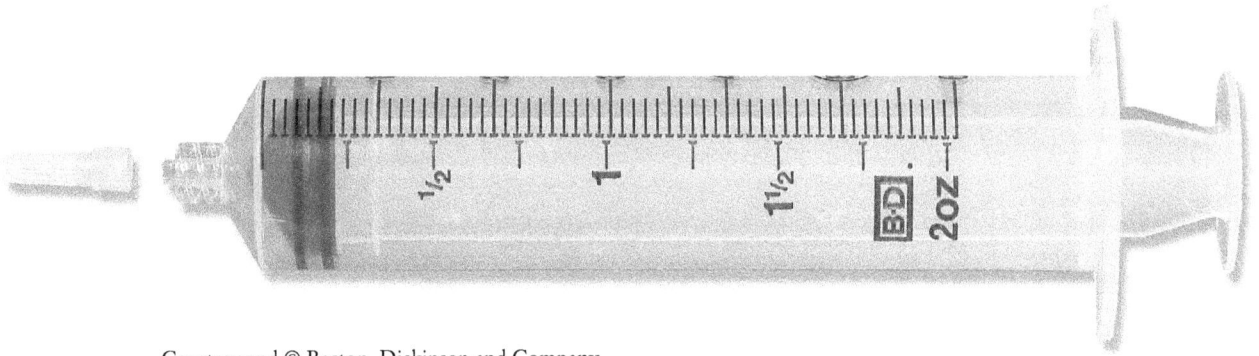

Courtesy and © Becton, Dickinson and Company

4. Draw a line to 13mls using the above syringe.

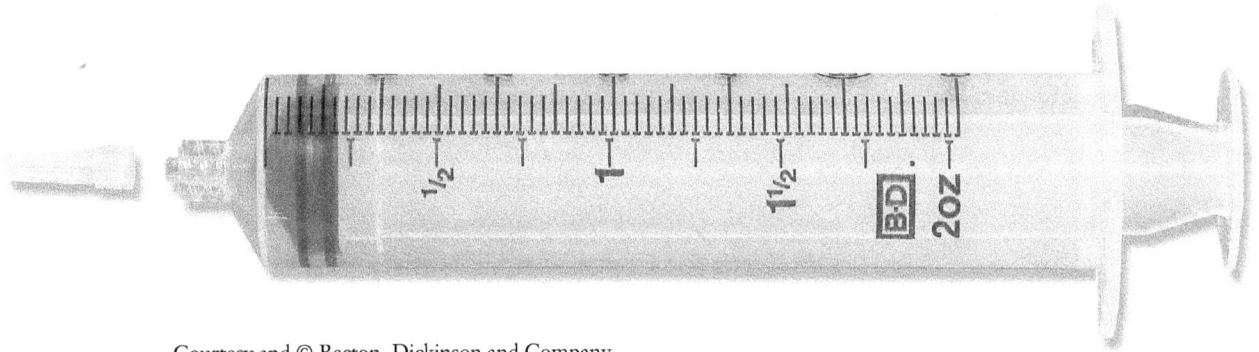

Courtesy and © Becton, Dickinson and Company

5. Draw a line to 37mls using the above syringe.

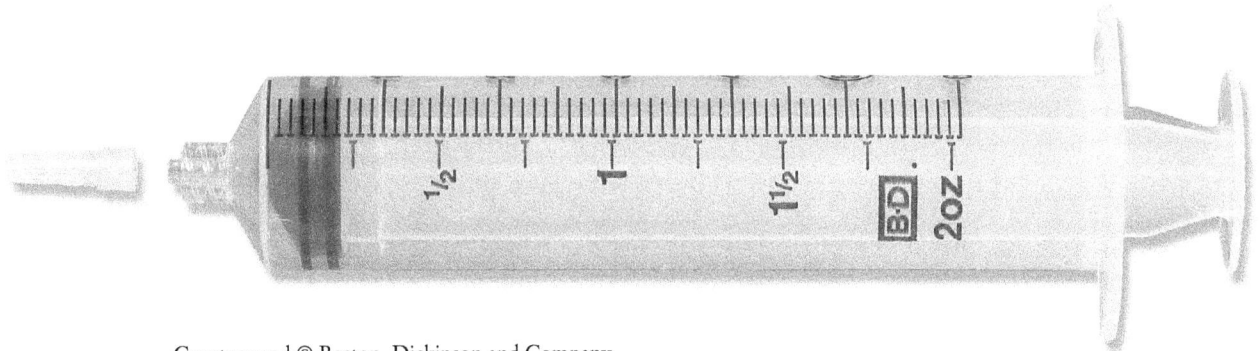

Courtesy and © Becton, Dickinson and Company

6. Draw a line to 6mls using the above syringe.

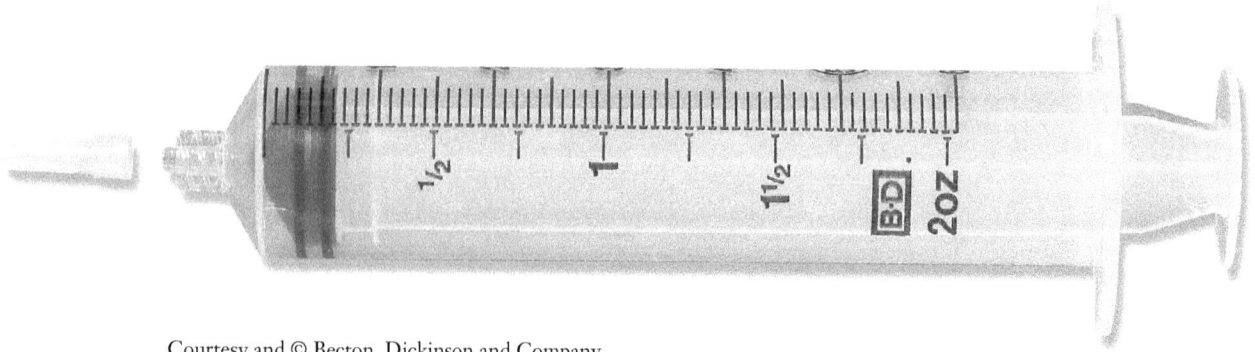

Courtesy and © Becton, Dickinson and Company

7. Draw a line to 43mls using the above syringe.

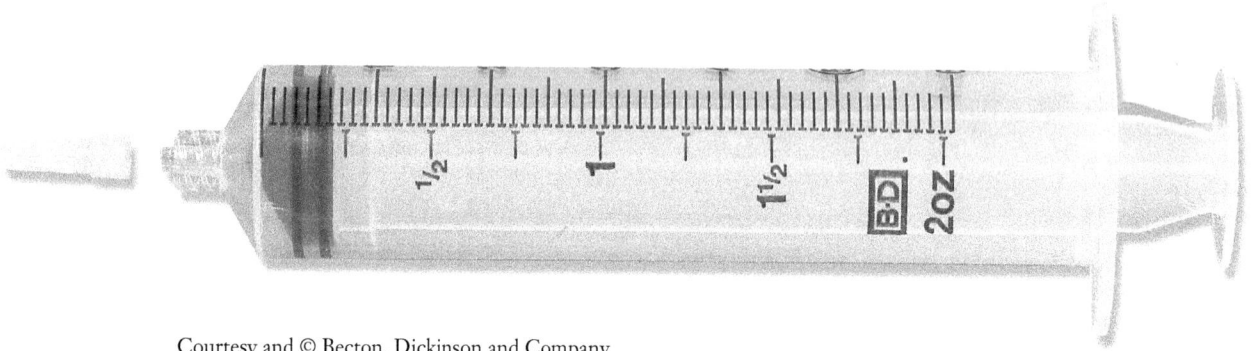

Courtesy and © Becton, Dickinson and Company

8. Draw a line to 32mls using the above syringe.

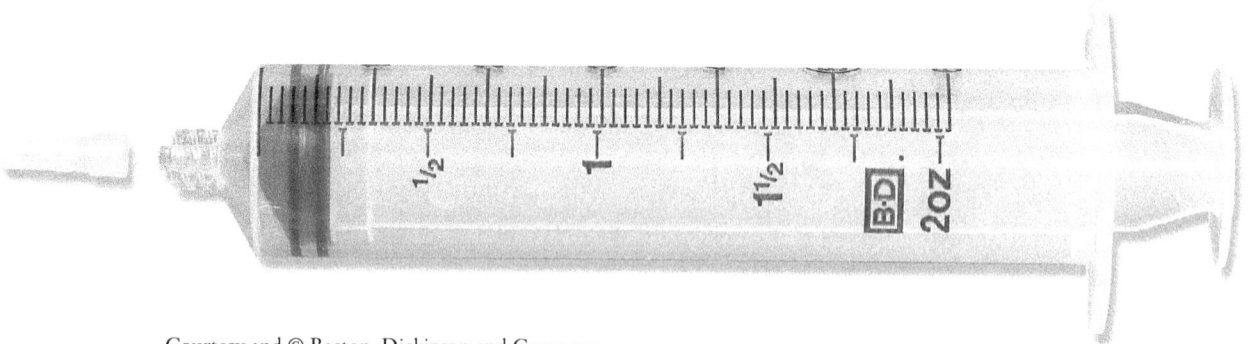

Courtesy and © Becton, Dickinson and Company

9. Draw a line to 56mls using the above syringe.

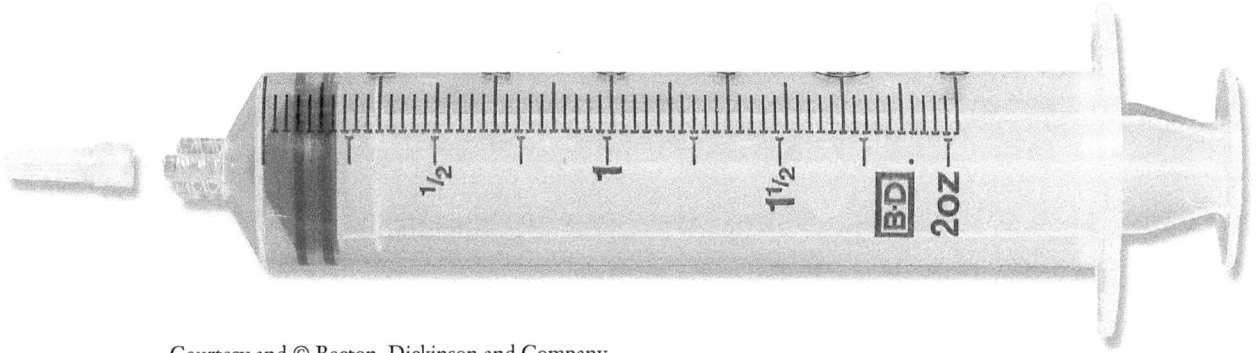

Courtesy and © Becton, Dickinson and Company

10. Draw a line to 3mls using the above syringe.

Lab 31: Alligations

OBJECTIVE

To understand how to calculate the needed amount of medication if two strengths are available.

INSTRUCTIONS

A patient comes into the pharmacy with a prescription that reads like the following:

Sample #1:

Ciprofloxacin 45% in 550 grams

Apply 1" ribbon q4hrs × 10d.

You have on the shelf Ciprofloxacin 35% and 65%.

You need to use both strengths to create strength of 45%. How do you do this? This is where alligations come into play.

Alligations are a math formula used in pharmacies to make special compounds for patients. These compounds can be made for a variety of reasons, but in this case we are assuming that the percentage that we need is not available. There are a variety of ways that a compound may be made.

Here is the break down of the steps needed to complete alligations:

Sample #1:

Highest %		Desired % – Lowest % = X
	Desired %	
Lowest %		Highest % – Desired % = X

			Parts Needed
65%		45% – 35% =	10
	45%		
35%		65% – 45% =	20

Total Parts = 10 + 20 = 30
30 Parts Total

In order to determine how many grams of 65% Ciprofloxacin is needed, we will calculate the following:

$$65\% = 550g \times \frac{10}{30} = 550g \times 0.33 = 181.5 \text{ g (hint: 10 divided by 30 = 0.33333 = 0.33)}$$

$$35\% = 550g \times \frac{20}{30} = 550g \times 0.67 = 368.5g$$

Conclusion:

In order to compound the following prescription the technician will need the following amounts from each of the stock supplied:

65% = 181.5 grams

35% = 268.5 grams

181.5 + 368.5 = 550 grams

The following items contain the stock strengths on the shelf pertaining to each prescription. Complete the calculations using the space provided.

1. 15% and 80%. How many mls of the 80% solution will be needed?

Dr. Phull, H	Dr. Diver, Skye	Dr. Bansal, S	Dr. Perez, C
Dr. Mundian, K	Dr. Virdee, S	Dr. Climber, R	Dr. Racer, C
Dr. Dhillon, S	Dr. Chana, C	Dr. McDonald, R	Dr. Radia, K

Bansal Urgent Care

Name: _____ Date: _____

Address: _____

RX

NS 65%

1 tsp bid x 30d

DAW ☐   Refill ②   MD _____   Lic. No : _____

DEA# _____

2. 25% and 46% solution. How many mls of the 25% solution is needed?

Dr. Phull, H	Dr. Diver, Skye	Dr. Bansal, S	Dr. Perez, C
Dr. Mundian, K	Dr. Virdee, S	Dr. Climber, R	Dr. Racer, C
Dr. Dhillon, S	Dr. Chana, C	Dr. McDonald, R	Dr. Radia, K

Bansal Urgent Care

Name: _____   Date: _____
Address: _____
RX

    amoxil 35%   XR

    T tsp bid X15d

DAW ☐   Refill ②   MD Radia K   Lic. No :
    DEA# _____

3. The pharmacy has ointment strength of 39% and 78% Vaseline. How much of each stock percentage is required?

Dr. Phull, H	Dr. Diver, Skye	Dr. Bansal, S	Dr. Perez, C
Dr. Mundian, K	Dr. Virdee, S	Dr. Climber, R	Dr. Racer, C
Dr. Dhillon, S	Dr. Chana, C	Dr. McDonald, R	Dr. Radia, K

Bansal Urgent Care

Name: _____   Date: _____
Address: _____
RX

    Vasoline 50%   #689

    AAA prn itching

DAW ☐   Refill ⑫   MD _____   Lic. No :
    DEA# _____

4. On the shelf you have 1.5% and 4%.

Dr. Phull, H	Dr. Diver, Skye	Dr. Bansal, S	Dr. Perez, C
Dr. Mundian, K	Dr. Virdee, S	Dr. Climber, R	Dr. Racer, C
Dr. Dhillon, S	Dr. Chana, C	Dr. McDonald, R	Dr. Radia, K

Bansal Urgent Care

Name: _____ Date: _____
Address: _____
RX

NTG 3.5% ung #50
unt

DAW ☐   Refill NR   MD Climber, R   Lic. No :
DEA#

5. On the shelf you have 50g of 7% and 25% cocoa butter. How do you fill this prescription?

Dr. Phull, H	Dr. Diver, Skye	Dr. Bansal, S	Dr. Perez, C
Dr. Mundian, K	Dr. Virdee, S	Dr. Climber, R	Dr. Racer, C
Dr. Dhillon, S	Dr. Chana, C	Dr. McDonald, R	Dr. Radia, K

Bansal Urgent Care

Name: _____ Date: _____
Address: _____
RX

Lotion 15%
apply to dry skin prn

DAW ☐   Refill ②   MD Dhillon, S.   Lic. No :
DEA#

6. On hand there is a solution that has a volume of 805 mls with strength of 26%. What will the final volume be?

Dr. Phull, H	Dr. Diver, Skye	Dr. Bansal, S	Dr. Perez, C
Dr. Mundian, K	Dr. Virdee, S	Dr. Climber, R	Dr. Racer, C
Dr. Dhillon, S	Dr. Chana, C	Dr. McDonald, R	Dr. Radia, K

Bansal Urgent Care

Name: _____ Date: _____
Address: _____
RX

Calamine lotion #500mls
32% AAA qid

DAW ☐   Refill ⑧   MD _Phull, H._   Lic. No : _____
                      DEA# _____

7. On the shelf you have 3% and 8.6% solution; how many parts will be needed total?

Dr. Phull, H	Dr. Diver, Skye	Dr. Bansal, S	Dr. Perez, C
Dr. Mundian, K	Dr. Virdee, S	Dr. Climber, R	Dr. Racer, C
Dr. Dhillon, S	Dr. Chana, C	Dr. McDonald, R	Dr. Radia, K

Bansal Urgent Care

Name: _____ Date: _____
Address: _____
RX

Tyco #3 6%
1-2 tsp q 4-6 hrs prn

DAW ☐   Refill _____   MD _____   Lic. No : _____
                      DEA# _____

8. How many milliliters of aloe vera should be added to 398 gm of calamine lotion that already contains 20% of aloe vera to compound a product that has 80% of aloe vera?

Dr. Phull, H	Dr. Diver, Skye	Dr. Bansal, S	Dr. Perez, C
Dr. Mundian, K	Dr. Virdee, S	Dr. Climber, R	
Dr. Dhillon, S	Dr. Chana, C	Dr. McDonald, R	

Bansal Urgent Care

Name: _____ Date: _____
Address: _____
RX

   Nystatin 35% #30g
      AAA uol

DAW ☐   Refill ②   MD *Bansal*   Lic. No :
                       DEA# _____

9. Available is 2.5% and 10%. How many mls of each is needed to make 250mls?

Dr. Phull, H	Dr. Diver, Skye	Dr. Bansal, S	Dr. Perez, C
Dr. Mundian, K	Dr. Virdee, S	Dr. Climber, R	Dr. Racer, C
Dr. Dhillon, S	Dr. Chana, C	Dr. McDonald, R	Dr. Radia, K

Bansal Urgent Care

Name: _____ Date: _____
Address: _____
RX

   Tegretal 4% #25mls
      T tbsp qam

DAW ☐   Refill ⑫   MD *Bansal*   Lic. No :
                       DEA# _____

10. You have on stock 15% and 50%. How much stock strength is needed?

Dr. Phull, H	Dr. Diver, Skye	Dr. Bansal, S	Dr. Perez, C
Dr. Mundian, K	Dr. Virdee, S	Dr. Climber, R	Dr. Racer, C
Dr. Dhillon, S	Dr. Chana, C	Dr. McDonald, R	Dr. Radia, K

Bansal Urgent Care

Name: _____ Date: _____
Address: _____
RX

Lamisel 29% Qty: 500g
AAA 9am + 8pm

DAW ☐   Refill ②   MD Diver, Skye   Lic. No :
DEA#

11. The stock on the shelf consists of 15% and 55% ointment. How many parts is needed in total?

Dr. Phull, H	Dr. Diver, Skye	Dr. Bansal, S	Dr. Perez, C
Dr. Mundian, K	Dr. Virdee, S	Dr. Climber, R	Dr. Racer, C
Dr. Dhillon, S	Dr. Chana, C	Dr. McDonald, R	Dr. Radia, K

Bansal Urgent Care

Name: _____ Date: _____
Address: _____
RX

Ketaconazole 25% #50ml
apply to infection qid

DAW ☐   Refill ②   MD Mundian, K.   Lic. No :
DEA#

12. Motrin 12% and 50% is on the shelf. How long will this prescription last?

Dr. Phull, H	Dr. Diver, Skye	Dr. Bansal, S	Dr. Perez, C
Dr. Mundian, K	Dr. Virdee, S	Dr. Climber, R	Dr. Racer, C
Dr. Dhillon, S	Dr. Chana, C	Dr. McDonald, R	Dr. Radia, K

Bansal Urgent Care

Name: _____ Date: _____

Address: _____

RX

Motrin 35%   #60 ml

T-ii tsp q4hrs prn back pain

DAW ☐   Refill ①   MD Chana, Ch.   Lic. No :

DEA#

13. Lidocaine 2.5% and 6.5% are on the shelf. How many grams of 6.5% is needed?

Dr. Phull, H	Dr. Diver, Skye	Dr. Bansal, S	Dr. Perez, C
Dr. Mundian, K	Dr. Virdee, S	Dr. Climber, R	Dr. Racer, C
Dr. Dhillon, S	Dr. Chana, C	Dr. McDonald, R	Dr. Radia, K

Bansal Urgent Care

Name: _____ Date: _____

Address: _____

RX

Lidocaine 5% #50g

ud.

DAW ☐   Refill Ø   MD McDonald, R   Lic. No :

DEA#

14. Paxil 88% and 55% are on the shelf. Mix accordingly.

Dr. Phull, H	Dr. Diver, Skye	Dr. Bansal, S	Dr. Perez, C
Dr. Mundian, K	Dr. Virdee, S	Dr. Climber, R	Dr. Racer, C
Dr. Dhillon, S	Dr. Chana, C	Dr. McDonald, R	Dr. Radia, K

Bansal Urgent Care

Name: _____   Date: _____
Address: _____
RX

   Paxil 78%   #250mls

      II mls qam + qpm #60d

DAW ☐   Refill _____   MD _Racer, C_____   Lic. No : _____
                          DEA# _____

15. Nystatin 20% and 45% is on the shelf. The patient is waiting for his prescription; complete the math as quickly as possible.

Dr. Phull, H	Dr. Diver, Skye	Dr. Bansal, S	Dr. Perez, C
Dr. Mundian, K	Dr. Virdee, S	Dr. Climber, R	
Dr. Dhillon, S	Dr. Chana, C	Dr. McDonald, R	

Bansal Urgent Care

Name: _____   Date: _____
Address: _____
RX

      Nystatin 35% #30g
          AAA ud

DAW ☐   Refill ②   MD _Bansal_____   Lic. No : _____
                          DEA# _____

Appendix

Adventure Pharmacy

Patient Name	AKA:		Sex: M / F		
Patient Address			Allergies:		
Patient DOB	Note:		Telephone #		
Insurance Name	Group: Relation:		ID #		
Date	Name, Strength of Medication	Directions	QTY DS	Physician	Refills Remaining
			QTY: Quantity to be Dispensed EDS: Estimated Day Supply		

Adventure Pharmacy

Patient Name	AKA:		Sex: M / F		
Patient Address			Allergies:		
Patient DOB	Note:		Telephone #		
Insurance Name	Group: Relation:		ID #		
Date	Name, Strength of Medication	Directions	QTY DS	Physician	Refills Remaining
			QTY: Quantity to be Dispensed EDS: Estimated Day Supply		

Adventure Pharmacy

Patient Name	AKA:		Sex: M / F			
Patient Address			Allergies:			
Patient DOB	Note:		Telephone #			
Insurance Name	Group: Relation:		ID #			
Date	Name, Strength of Medication	Directions	QTY DS		Physician	Refills Remaining
			QTY: Quantity to be Dispensed EDS: Estimated Day Supply			

Adventure Pharmacy

Patient Name	AKA:		Sex: M / F			
Patient Address			Allergies:			
Patient DOB	Note:		Telephone #			
Insurance Name	Group: Relation:		ID #			
Date	Name, Strength of Medication	Directions	QTY DS		Physician	Refills Remaining
			QTY: Quantity to be Dispensed EDS: Estimated Day Supply			

Adventure Pharmacy

Patient Name	AKA:		Sex: M / F			
Patient Address			Allergies:			
Patient DOB	Note:		Telephone #			
Insurance Name	Group:	Relation:	ID #			
Date	Name, Strength of Medication	Directions	QTY DS		Physician	Refills Remaining
			QTY: Quantity to be Dispensed EDS: Estimated Day Supply			

Adventure Pharmacy

Patient Name	AKA:		Sex: M / F			
Patient Address			Allergies:			
Patient DOB	Note:		Telephone #			
Insurance Name	Group:	Relation:	ID #			
Date	Name, Strength of Medication	Directions	QTY DS		Physician	Refills Remaining
			QTY: Quantity to be Dispensed EDS: Estimated Day Supply			

Adventure Pharmacy

Patient Name	AKA:		Sex: M / F			
Patient Address			Allergies:			
Patient DOB	Note:		Telephone #			
Insurance Name	Group:	Relation:	ID #			
Date	Name, Strength of Medication	Directions	QTY DS		Physician	Refills Remaining
QTY: Quantity to be Dispensed EDS: Estimated Day Supply						

Adventure Pharmacy

Patient Name	AKA:		Sex: M / F			
Patient Address			Allergies:			
Patient DOB	Note:		Telephone #			
Insurance Name	Group:	Relation:	ID #			
Date	Name, Strength of Medication	Directions	QTY DS		Physician	Refills Remaining
QTY: Quantity to be Dispensed EDS: Estimated Day Supply						

Adventure Pharmacy

Patient Name	AKA:			Sex: M / F		
Patient Address				Allergies:		
Patient DOB	Note:			Telephone #		
Insurance Name	Group: Relation:			ID #		
Date	Name, Strength of Medication	Directions	QTY DS	Physician	Refills Remaining	
			QTY: Quantity to be Dispensed EDS: Estimated Day Supply			

Adventure Pharmacy

Patient Name	AKA:			Sex: M / F		
Patient Address				Allergies:		
Patient DOB	Note:			Telephone #		
Insurance Name	Group: Relation:			ID #		
Date	Name, Strength of Medication	Directions	QTY DS	Physician	Refills Remaining	
			QTY: Quantity to be Dispensed EDS: Estimated Day Supply			

ADVENTURE HOSPITAL
TPN PHARMACY ORDER

Patient Name   _____

Allergies _____

MR # _____

Calculate the amount of grams needed per day for the standard formula; calculate the ml to be given per liter for the additives. Complete one TPN pharmacy order for each day per patient

Indication for TPN: _____ Wt: _____

Route: ☐ Central Line (CL)   ☐ Peripheral Line (PL)

Date: _____

Flow Rate _____ ml/hr, Total ml/day _____, Total L/day _____

Standard Formula:	Recommended Dosage	Per Day
Amino Acids	4GM/kg	_____ GM
Dextrose	1.5GM/kg	_____ GM
Lipids	1GM/kg	_____ GM

Additives (available stock):		Per Dose	Per Dose
KCl	(40mEq/50ml)	_____ mEq	_____ ml
NaAcetate	(40mEq/ml)	_____ mEq	_____ ml
CaGluconate	(45mEq/ml)	_____ mEq	_____ ml
MgSO$_4$	(5mEq/2.5ml)	_____ mEq	_____ ml
Multivit Conc.	———	_____ ml	_____ ml
Zn	(1mg/ml)	_____ mg	_____ ml
Cu	(0.4mg/ml)	_____ mg	_____ ml
Mn	(4mg/3ml)	_____ mg	_____ ml
Cr	(4mcg/ml)	_____ mg	_____ ml
Insulin		_____ U	_____ ml

STANDARD PHARMACY ORDERS:
Always compound TPN / IV using aseptic technique

Pharmacy Technician Name: _____

Pharmacy Technician Signature: _____

Date: _____

ADVENTURE HOSPITAL
TPN PHARMACY ORDER

Patient Name _____

Allergies _____

MR # _____

Calculate the amount of grams needed per day for the standard formula; calculate the ml to be given per liter for the additives. Complete one TPN pharmacy order for each day per patient

Indication for TPN: _____ Wt: _____

Route: ☐ Central Line (CL)   ☐ Peripheral Line (PL)

Date: _____

Flow Rate _____ ml/hr, Total ml/day _____, Total L/day _____

Standard Formula:	Recommended Dosage	Per Day
Amino Acids	4GM/kg	_____ GM
Dextrose	1.5GM/kg	_____ GM
Lipids	1GM/kg	_____ GM

Additives (available stock):		Per Dose	Per Dose
KCl	(40mEq/50ml)	_____ mEq	_____ ml
NaAcetate	(40mEq/ml)	_____ mEq	_____ ml
CaGluconate	(45mEq/ml)	_____ mEq	_____ ml
$MgSO_4$	(5mEq/2.5ml)	_____ mEq	_____ ml
Multivit Conc.	———	_____ ml	_____ ml
Zn	(1mg/ml)	_____ mg	_____ ml
Cu	(0.4mg/ml)	_____ mg	_____ ml
Mn	(4mg/3ml)	_____ mg	_____ ml
Cr	(4mcg/ml)	_____ mg	_____ ml
Insulin		_____ U	_____ ml

STANDARD PHARMACY ORDERS:
Always compound TPN / IV using aseptic technique

Pharmacy Technician Name: _____

Pharmacy Technician Signature: _____

Date: _____

ADVENTURE HOSPITAL
TPN PHARMACY ORDER

Patient Name _____

Allergies _____

MR # _____

Calculate the amount of grams needed per day for the standard formula; calculate the ml to be given per liter for the additives. Complete one TPN pharmacy order for each day per patient

Indication for TPN: _____ Wt: _____

Route: ☐ Central Line (CL) ☐ Peripheral Line (PL)

Date: _____

Flow Rate _____ ml/hr, Total ml/day _____, Total L/day _____

Standard Formula:	Recommended Dosage	Per Day
Amino Acids	4GM/kg	_____ GM
Dextrose	1.5GM/kg	_____ GM
Lipids	1GM/kg	_____ GM

Additives (available stock):		Per Dose	Per Dose
KCl	(40mEq/50ml)	_____ mEq	_____ ml
NaAcetate	(40mEq/ml)	_____ mEq	_____ ml
CaGluconate	(45mEq/ml)	_____ mEq	_____ ml
$MgSO_4$	(5mEq/2.5ml)	_____ mEq	_____ ml
Multivit Conc.	———	_____ ml	_____ ml
Zn	(1mg/ml)	_____ mg	_____ ml
Cu	(0.4mg/ml)	_____ mg	_____ ml
Mn	(4mg/3ml)	_____ mg	_____ ml
Cr	(4mcg/ml)	_____ mg	_____ ml
Insulin		_____ U	_____ ml

STANDARD PHARMACY ORDERS:
Always compound TPN / IV using aseptic technique

Pharmacy Technician Name: _____

Pharmacy Technician Signature: _____

Date: _____

ADVENTURE HOSPITAL
TPN PHARMACY ORDER

Patient Name _____

Allergies _____

MR # _____

Calculate the amount of grams needed per day for the standard formula; calculate the ml to be given per liter for the additives. Complete one TPN pharmacy order for each day per patient

Indication for TPN: _____ Wt: _____

Route: ☐ Central Line (CL)   ☐ Peripheral Line (PL)

Date: _____

Flow Rate _____ ml/hr, Total ml/day _____, Total L/day _____

Standard Formula:		Recommended Dosage	Per Day	
Amino Acids		4GM/kg	_____	GM
Dextrose		1.5GM/kg	_____	GM
Lipids		1GM/kg	_____	GM

Additives (available stock):		Per Dose		Per Dose	
KCl	(40mEq/50ml)	_____	mEq	_____	ml
NaAcetate	(40mEq/ml)	_____	mEq	_____	ml
CaGluconate	(45mEq/ml)	_____	mEq	_____	ml
$MgSO_4$	(5mEq/2.5ml)	_____	mEq	_____	ml
Multivit Conc.	_____	_____	ml	_____	ml
Zn	(1mg/ml)	_____	mg	_____	ml
Cu	(0.4mg/ml)	_____	mg	_____	ml
Mn	(4mg/3ml)	_____	mg	_____	ml
Cr	(4mcg/ml)	_____	mg	_____	ml
Insulin		_____	U	_____	ml

STANDARD PHARMACY ORDERS:
Always compound TPN / IV using aseptic technique

Pharmacy Technician Name: _____

Pharmacy Technician Signature: _____

Date: _____

ADVENTURE HOSPITAL
TPN PHARMACY ORDER

Patient Name _____

Allergies _____

MR # _____

Calculate the amount of grams needed per day for the standard formula; calculate the ml to be given per liter for the additives. Complete one TPN pharmacy order for each day per patient

Indication for TPN: _____ Wt: _____

Route: ☐ Central Line (CL) ☐ Peripheral Line (PL)

Date: _____

Flow Rate _____ ml/hr, Total ml/day _____, Total L/day _____

Standard Formula:	Recommended Dosage	Per Day
Amino Acids	4GM/kg	_____ GM
Dextrose	1.5GM/kg	_____ GM
Lipids	1GM/kg	_____ GM

Additives (available stock):		Per Dose	Per Dose
KCl	(40mEq/50ml)	_____ mEq	_____ ml
NaAcetate	(40mEq/ml)	_____ mEq	_____ ml
CaGluconate	(45mEq/ml)	_____ mEq	_____ ml
$MgSO_4$	(5mEq/2.5ml)	_____ mEq	_____ ml
Multivit Conc.	———	_____ ml	_____ ml
Zn	(1mg/ml)	_____ mg	_____ ml
Cu	(0.4mg/ml)	_____ mg	_____ ml
Mn	(4mg/3ml)	_____ mg	_____ ml
Cr	(4mcg/ml)	_____ mg	_____ ml
Insulin		_____ U	_____ ml

STANDARD PHARMACY ORDERS:
Always compound TPN / IV using aseptic technique

Pharmacy Technician Name: _____

Pharmacy Technician Signature: _____

Date: _____

ADVENTURE HOSPITAL
TPN PHARMACY ORDER

Patient Name _____

Allergies _____

MR # _____

Calculate the amount of grams needed per day for the standard formula; calculate the ml to be given per liter for the additives. Complete one TPN pharmacy order for each day per patient

Indication for TPN: _____ Wt: _____

Route: ☐ Central Line (CL)   ☐ Peripheral Line (PL)

Date: _____

Flow Rate _____ ml/hr, Total ml/day _____, Total L/day _____

Standard Formula:		Recommended Dosage	Per Day
Amino Acids		4GM/kg	_____ GM
Dextrose		1.5GM/kg	_____ GM
Lipids		1GM/kg	_____ GM

Additives (available stock):		Per Dose	Per Dose
KCl	(40mEq/50ml)	_____ mEq	_____ ml
NaAcetate	(40mEq/ml)	_____ mEq	_____ ml
CaGluconate	(45mEq/ml)	_____ mEq	_____ ml
MgSO$_4$	(5mEq/2.5ml)	_____ mEq	_____ ml
Multivit Conc.	———	_____ ml	_____ ml
Zn	(1mg/ml)	_____ mg	_____ ml
Cu	(0.4mg/ml)	_____ mg	_____ ml
Mn	(4mg/3ml)	_____ mg	_____ ml
Cr	(4mcg/ml)	_____ mg	_____ ml
Insulin		_____ U	_____ ml

STANDARD PHARMACY ORDERS:
Always compound TPN / IV using aseptic technique

Pharmacy Technician Name: _____

Pharmacy Technician Signature: _____

Date: _____

ADVENTURE HOSPITAL
TPN PHARMACY ORDER

Patient Name _____

Allergies _____

MR # _____

Calculate the amount of grams needed per day for the standard formula; calculate the ml to be given per liter for the additives. Complete one TPN pharmacy order for each day per patient

Indication for TPN: _____ Wt: _____

Route: ☐ Central Line (CL) ☐ Peripheral Line (PL)

Date: _____

Flow Rate _____ ml/hr, Total ml/day _____, Total L/day _____

Standard Formula:	Recommended Dosage	Per Day
Amino Acids	4GM/kg	_____ GM
Dextrose	1.5GM/kg	_____ GM
Lipids	1GM/kg	_____ GM

Additives (available stock):		Per Dose	Per Dose
KCl	(40mEq/50ml)	_____ mEq	_____ ml
NaAcetate	(40mEq/ml)	_____ mEq	_____ ml
CaGluconate	(45mEq/ml)	_____ mEq	_____ ml
$MgSO_4$	(5mEq/2.5ml)	_____ mEq	_____ ml
Multivit Conc.	———	_____ ml	_____ ml
Zn	(1mg/ml)	_____ mg	_____ ml
Cu	(0.4mg/ml)	_____ mg	_____ ml
Mn	(4mg/3ml)	_____ mg	_____ ml
Cr	(4mcg/ml)	_____ mg	_____ ml
Insulin		_____ U	_____ ml

STANDARD PHARMACY ORDERS:
Always compound TPN / IV using aseptic technique

Pharmacy Technician Name: _____

Pharmacy Technician Signature: _____

Date: _____

Authorization for Treatment

Patient Name _____
                              Last   First   Middle

Mailing Address _____

Subscriber ID_____ Patient Date of Birth _____

Sex   M   F   Relationship to subscriber _____

Subscriber Phone Number _____

Description of Diagnosis _____

Medical Justification:

_____

_____

_____

Drug Name and Strength	Directions	Quantity / Charge	NDC #	Initials of Provider / Title

Name of Pharmacy_____

Address_____

Phone Number _____

Provider Signature _____ Date_____

Authorization for Treatment

Patient Name _____

                         Last   First   Middle

Mailing Address _____

Subscriber ID_____ Patient Date of Birth _____

Sex M F   Relationship to subscriber _____

Subscriber Phone Number _____

Description of Diagnosis _____

Medical Justification:

_____

_____

_____

Drug Name and Strength	Directions	Quantity / Charge	NDC #	Initials of Provider / Title

Name of Pharmacy_____

Address_____

Phone Number _____

Provider Signature _____ Date_____

Authorization for Treatment

Patient Name _____
                         Last   First   Middle

Mailing Address _____

Subscriber ID_____   Patient Date of Birth _____

Sex   M   F   Relationship to subscriber _____

Subscriber Phone Number _____

Description of Diagnosis _____

Medical Justification:

_____

_____

_____

Drug Name and Strength	Directions	Quantity / Charge	NDC #	Initials of Provider / Title

Name of Pharmacy_____

Address_____

Phone Number _____

Provider Signature _____   Date_____

Authorization for Treatment

Patient Name _____

                     Last   First   Middle

Mailing Address _____

Subscriber ID_____   Patient Date of Birth _____

Sex M F   Relationship to subscriber _____

Subscriber Phone Number _____

Description of Diagnosis _____

Medical Justification:

_____

_____

_____

Drug Name and Strength	Directions	Quantity / Charge	NDC #	Initials of Provider / Title

Name of Pharmacy _____

Address_____

Phone Number _____

Provider Signature _____   Date_____

Authorization for Treatment

Patient Name _____
                                           Last   First   Middle

Mailing Address _____

Subscriber ID_____ Patient Date of Birth _____

Sex M F   Relationship to subscriber _____

Subscriber Phone Number _____

Description of Diagnosis _____

Medical Justification:

_____

_____

_____

Drug Name and Strength	Directions	Quantity / Charge	NDC #	Initials of Provider / Title

Name of Pharmacy _____

Address_____

Phone Number _____

Provider Signature _____ Date_____

Authorization for Treatment

Patient Name _____

                      Last   First   Middle

Mailing Address _____

Subscriber ID_____ Patient Date of Birth _____

Sex M F   Relationship to subscriber _____

Subscriber Phone Number _____

Description of Diagnosis _____

Medical Justification:

_____

_____

_____

Drug Name and Strength	Directions	Quantity / Charge	NDC #	Initials of Provider / Title

Name of Pharmacy_____

Address_____

Phone Number _____

Provider Signature _____ Date_____

Authorization for Treatment

Patient Name _____
                           Last   First   Middle

Mailing Address _____

Subscriber ID _____   Patient Date of Birth _____

Sex M F   Relationship to subscriber _____

Subscriber Phone Number _____

Description of Diagnosis _____

Medical Justification:

_____

_____

_____

Drug Name and Strength	Directions	Quantity / Charge	NDC #	Initials of Provider / Title

Name of Pharmacy _____

Address_____

Phone Number _____

Provider Signature _____   Date_____

Index

www.ingramcontent.com/pod-product-compliance
Lightning Source LLC
Chambersburg PA
CBHW080913220326
41598CB00034B/5557